Stressed Out

About Your First Year of Nursing

Patricia A. Duclos-Miller, MS, RN, CNA, BC

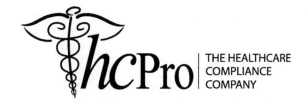

hcPro | THE HEALTHCARE
COMPLIANCE
COMPANY

Stressed Out About Your First Year of Nursing is published by HCPro, Inc.

Copyright ©2006 HCPro, Inc.

ISBN-13: 978-1-57839-931-4
ISBN-10: 1-57839-931-9

HCPro, Inc., provides information resources for the healthcare industry.

HCPro, Inc., is not affiliated in any way with The Joint Commission, which owns the JCAHO and Joint Commission trademarks.

MAGNET™, MAGNET RECOGNITION PROGRAM®, and ANCC MAGNET RECOGNITION® are trademarks of the American Nurses Credentialing Center (ANCC). The products and services of HCPro, Inc. and The Greeley Company are neither sponsored nor endorsed by the ANCC.

Patricia A. Duclos-Miller, MS, RN, CNA, BC, Author   Mike Mirabello, Senior Graphic Artist
Amanda Waddell, Associate Editor   Jean St. Pierre, Director of Operations
Emily Sheahan, Group Publisher   Darren Kelly, Books Production Supervisor
Shane Katz, Cover Designer   Matthew Kurht, Copyeditor

Cover illustration by Graham Smith, ArtMasters

Advice given is general. Readers should consult professional counsel for specific legal, ethical, or clinical questions. Arrangements can be made for quantity discounts. For more information, contact

HCPro, Inc.
P.O. Box 1168
Marblehead, MA 01945
Telephone: 800/650-6787 or 781/639-1872
Fax: 781/639-2982
E-mail: *customerservice@hcpro.com*

Visit the Stressed Out Web site for more information: *www.stressedoutnurses.com*

REV. 08/2007
21273

Dedication

This book is dedicated to all of the new nurses joining us in making a difference in our patients' lives. You are all entering the noblest profession—one that balances head, heart, and hands.

Contents

List of figures

Chapter 1

Chapter 2

Chapter 3

Chapter 4

Chapter 5

Chapter 6

Chapter 7

Chapter 8

Chapter 9

Chapter 10

How to use this book

What if there was a book that explained complex nursing topics in an easy-to-understand manner and in an accessible format? That's the premise behind the *Stressed Out...*series. Solid references with a bit of a sense of humor and the understanding that a lighthearted approach to learning makes the whole thing more enjoyable.

To help you navigate through the book, you will find the following icons highlighting a particular passage:

 Don't forget: A little reminder about something of importance.

 Ask: This icon directs you to search for further information from an individual or organization.

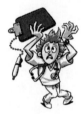 **Don't panic:** Take a deep breath and relax. Here is a little reassurance.

 Fact: Highlights a statistic or truth.

Tip: A bit of inside information, a hint, or helpful advice.

 Watch out: Word to the wise; this is a warning.

 Click: This icon refers you to a helpful Web site, where you may find further information on the topic.

Happy Nursing! Now you're ready to get started.

About the author

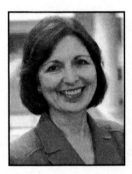

Patricia A. Duclos-Miller, MS, RN, CNA, BC

Patricia A. Duclos-Miller, MS, RN, CNA, BC, is currently a full-time associate professor in nursing at Capital Community College in Hartford, CT. In addition to this position, she is a consultant for the Kelsco Consulting Group in Chesire, CT, a special lecturer for the University of Connecticut's graduate nursing program, and a per diem supervisor at Bristol Hospital, CT.

During her 32 years in nursing, Duclos-Miller has served in a variety of roles, including staff nurse in the specialties of medical/surgical nursing, obstetrical nursing, and neonatal intensive care. She has also served as a nurse adminis-trator in the performance improvement, acute, home healthcare, and long-term care settings. Duclos-Miller is a recognized speaker on contemporary nursing topics such as quality, team building, and documentation issues.

In addition, Duclos-Miller has served in key leadership positions for pro-fessional organizations and is the author of the HCPro book *Managing Documentation Risk: A Guide for Nurse Managers.* She has also spoken about documentation on several HCPro audioconferences and is a contributor to the newsletter *Strategies for Nurse Managers.*

Duclos-Miller is a registered nurse and is board certified by the American Nurses Credentialing Center (ANCC) in nursing administration.

Acknowledgements

I am grateful for the nurse researchers who continue to make a contribution in helping us understand and change our profession for the better. I would like to express my appreciation to my editors, Rebecca Hendren and Amanda Waddell, for their capable and professional support and guidance. I am also thankful for my friends and colleagues for taking the time to listen and give their suggestions for the book, especially Liza Malchiodi, Judy Conway, Regina McNamara, Diane Perreault, Rosemary Hathaway, and Karen Ragaisis. A special thanks to Lien Tran for her assistance in my research.

Finally, thank you to all of the recent graduate nurses who were willing to share their experiences with me.

Introduction

You made it!

You made it through nursing school and you passed your NCLEX® exam. Your dreams of becoming a nurse are finally coming true. Before you step into this exciting new role, you'll need some sound advice on how to survive your first year in the profession. This valuable advice will help you avoid becoming one of the many new graduates who have difficulty managing their grueling first year and leave nursing altogether. You want to come out a winner and you can—just reach inside and believe in yourself. You've made it this far!

Stressed Out About Your First Year as a Nurse will help you successfully navigate through your first year and show you that you are not alone in your fears and self-doubt. You will learn that most new graduates have experienced the same emotions and frustrations as you—and survived!

This book will also give you sound advice on

- Why nursing today is so demanding, and how to survive these demands

- What to expect during orientation and how to ensure you get what you need to become a great nurse

- What the common causes of stress in nursing are and how to handle them

- How to manage the transition from student nurse to new graduate

- Understanding the stages of competence and determining your current stage

- How to handle "bullying," or horizontal violence

- Survival skills for today's nurse

- How to avoid legal pitfalls and stay out of trouble

So read on and learn how to make it through the most challenging year for every nurse. You can do it with a little help from this book and from others who will support your success along the way. The nursing profession is waiting for you—get on board!

Part One

Before you can begin your career as an RN, you need to find the right job for you. This section covers how to land that perfect position and gives you all the job essentials you need to succeed.

Chapter 1

Before you start looking for your first job

Step one: Self-assessment—be honest but true to yourself

Before you begin your first job search you need to think about what you expect from nursing. In order to be successful in the profession, you will have to do a self-assessment first, and then apply for the right job.

In your self-assessment, ask yourself

- What do I want out of nursing?

- With what types of patients am I interested in working?

- What are my clinical interests?

- What size of organization and nursing unit best suits me?

- What are my likes and dislikes related to my potential job?

- What shift(s) can I realistically handle?

- Do I like a stable or constantly changing environment?

After you have answered these questions and developed a strong sense of who you are and what you are looking for, you can begin to determine what area of nursing best suits you—and vice versa. Here are some generalizations about the different types of nursing units to help you decide what type of nursing is best for you:

Intensive Care Unit (ICU): Do you like being a skilled technician? Do you have very good assessment and prioritization skills? Do you like to work with complex physiological patients and their families? Does the team work well together? How well do you tolerate stress?

Emergency Department (ED): Do you like working in a fast-paced environment? Can you handle unanticipated and ever-changing levels of acuity and diagnosis? Do you like to work with trauma patients? Can you handle death? Do you work well on a team? How well do you tolerate stress?

Medical unit: Do you like dealing with chronic diseases, chronic wounds, and diabetic management? How well could you deal with readmissions of the same patient?

Surgical unit: Do you like working with surgical wounds, post-operative care, and pain management? Do you like working with managed care? Do you like working with other professional members of the team, such as the physical therapist (PT), occupational therapist (OT), and speech language therapist (SLT)?

Geriatric unit: Do you like working with the elderly and getting to know them? Do you like having a predictable work day? Can you effectively monitor staff who are responsible for the direct care of the patient?

Behavioral health unit: Do you prefer process orientation to outcome orientation? Do you consider patient communication a higher priority than developing your technical skills?

Obstetric unit (OB)/Parent-child health unit: Do you like treating the same type of patient day in and day out? Do you like patient teaching and repetition?

Pediatric (PEDS) unit: Do you enjoy working with sick children and their families? Do you like patient teaching?

Tip: As you can see, each specialty is different—and each has its own challenges and rewards. You need to look carefully at which area fits your desired population of patients, desired level of disease management, communication style, and teaching skills. Be honest with yourself, and make a commitment to succeed and be happy in nursing.

Where do I look?

There are many ways to search for the perfect job. The media have expanded from print (newspaper advertisements, journals, and newsletters) to Web sites and online advertising. In addition, there are live events that you can attend to help you with your search.

You should attend at least two career fairs that are exclusively for nurses. In addition, attend the open houses of any potential employers. These events provide a wonderful opportunity for you to speak with staff and tour the facility.

Another way to find a job is through networking and word of mouth. When you belong to a professional organization, there are always job opportunities that have yet to be posted or advertised, but are discussed among members at the meetings.

How do I compare hospitals/organizations?

Quality indicators are now reportable to the public. There are many Web sites, such as *www.hospitalcompare.hhs.gov*, that will list the clinical quality indicators for each hospital, home health agency, and long-term care facility in the United States.

Watch out: On these sites, spend time looking at the organization's last JCAHO survey results, the last state/federal survey results, and some of the commercial "report cards" that are open to the public. These results will give you an idea of the organization's level of commitment to quality, especially in comparison to other organizations in the state and nation. And, with so many healthcare systems in financial crisis, make it a priority to find out about the financial security of the organization.

In addition to researching the organization as a whole, be sure to ask about the reputation of nursing leadership in the prospective organization. If you did your clinical work at the organization, you can do this by talking to nurses with whom you worked. If you are unfamiliar with the organization, have an informal chat with staff before your formal interview. Consider asking the following questions:

- What is the organization's leadership style?

- Do leaders promote nursing?

- Are they innovative and creative?

What is the ANCC Magnet Recognition Program®?

Over the years, nursing has defined itself as a profession with high standards. One of the highest standards for an organization committed to nursing and quality patient care is the achievement of the American Nurses Credentialing Center's (ANCC) Magnet Recognition Program®. As of 2006, less than 3% of hospitals in the United States have been awarded designation. Some of the key characteristics of designated hospitals are

- The nurse executive is visible, influential, credible, and responsive. The value of the professional nurse is apparent.

- The administrative team listens and responds to its employees. Administration also recognizes the value of nursing. Dollars are put into the nursing budget, rather than taken away.

- The nurse leader articulates the importance of nursing to the administrative team, medical staff, and community members.

- There is mutual respect among the nursing, medical, and administrative staff. The goal is optimal patient care.

- The clinical staff works in a supportive, autonomous environment.

- Nurses are encouraged to move and grow to reach their potential. Nurses are financially supported to attend local and national conferences in order to stay abreast of current nursing trends.

- Nurses are provided the resources needed to perform their job, such as new equipment, better staffing and assistive help. They are paid well.

- Even with the nursing shortage, there are enough nurses who are satisfied and empowered in their role. They provide excellent patient care (Upenieks 2002).

Designated facilities report higher patient satisfaction scores, achieve better patient outcomes, provide more nursing care at the bedside, and have higher retention rates than nondesignated organizations (Greiner and Hendrich 2006). For these reasons, pursuing employment at a designated facility may prove to be an attractive option.

Collective bargaining: What is it?

You may have heard the term "union" or collective bargaining. Collective bargaining may be defined as activities that occur between organized labor and the organization (your employer) that involve employee relations. An example of this is the discussion of a new formal written contract for those in a collective bargaining agreement.

There are many different collective-bargaining/union organizations across the country. They represent workers in almost all facets of the work world. Nurses are represented by some of the unions that also represent teachers, auto, and service workers. The hospital in which you are interested may have a nursing staff represented by a union such as the American Federation of Labor and Congress of Industrial Organizations (AFL-CIO), the Service Employee Industry Union (SEIU), or the United American Nurses (UAN). Or, the hospital may be using non-traditional collective-bargaining approaches that have emerged over the last few years.

 Tip: If you are seeking employment in an environment that relies on collective bargaining, you need to understand how the nurses are represented in the organization and ensure that the voice of nursing is being heard. The following are some common terms you may encounter:

Interest-based bargaining (IBB): a non-traditional approach to collective bargaining. IBB involves shared governance, and a collaborative problem-solving approach to workplace issues and nursing practice.

Center for American Nurses (CAN): an organizational member of the professional association, the American Nurses Association. The CAN represents the interests of nurses who are not formally part of a union. They encourage workplace advocacy as a means for the promotion of positive work environments.

United American Nurses (UAN): a traditional collective-bargaining unit that is affiliated with the American Nurses Association, but is a member of the AFL-CIO.

Traditional collective bargaining: a regulated collective-bargaining unit or union. The goal is to help its members gain control over practice, economics in the healthcare industry, and other issues that may impede the quality of patient care (Zerwekh and Claborn 2006).

Watch out: If you plan to join an organization that is affiliated with a union, you need to understand not only what membership in the union entails, but what is expected of you as a union member. For example, union membership requires payment of annual dues and participation in actions such as strikes.

Figure 1.1: Unions—To join or not to join

Benefits	Drawbacks
• Better wages • Better benefits • Better staffing ratios • Help with grievances • Solidarity • Protection from poor working conditions	• No voice as an individual • Difficult to get rid of poor-performing nurses • Jobs and prime vacation time awarded to senior staff • Dues • Strikes

---

Job search essentials

Résumés: The key to getting the best job out there

Presentation is everything. Remember the phrase, "It's all in the packaging"? When it comes to your résumé, that phrase couldn't be more true. Your goal is to impress anyone who may see your résumé come across their desk. A well constructed résumé will set itself apart from the dozens of others that your potential employer sees on a daily basis.

Tip: Use the correct font, usually 12-point type, Arial or Helvetica font. Use a quality paper in a neutral color (white or cream). Also, use a manila mailing envelope that is 8.5 x 11 inches, and that does not require you to fold your résumé. You want the finished résumé to look professional and show the employer that you are a conscientious person who pays attention to detail.

Don't forget: When preparing your résumé, include the following:

- **Name, address, and phone number.** This should appear at the top of the page. Most people center this information, but there are impressive résumés that use the right- or left-justified format. As you will be listing your contact information, be sure your answering machine or voicemail recording sounds professional—no hard rock, funny introduction, or cute children on the recording. Remember that this is your potential employer's first contact with you. You want to project a good impression and show that you are serious about this job. You should also consider establishing a new e-mail address for your job search, especially if your current address is something like fairygodmother@abc.com.

- **Job titles.** These should be clear and understandable to the human resources department and hiring manager. Do not use abbreviations unless you also spell them out, e.g., "PCA (Patient Care Associate)."

- **Company names and dates,** which are an important indicator of your work history. List the month and year in which you began each job, as well as the month and year in which you ended your employment. Remember to list your part-time and summer work positions, as they illustrate your work ethic and project the image that you were able to manage school and work. Under each job, list the **job duties** that were required for the position. You can also highlight your achievements and demonstrate if you exceeded the expected job requirements.

- **Volunteer work,** if you have participated in a substantial amount. This shows that you have initiative, a commitment to civic duty, self-motivation, and leadership and communication skills.

- **Certification,** an important aspect of the nursing profession. Be sure to list all areas of certification on your résumé, including your CPR (cardiopulmonary resuscitation) certification and any other related certifications.

- **Education,** listed by the highest level reached first. This section becomes less important as you gain experience as a registered nurse. Once you have acquired several years of applicable work history, you should put education after your employment history.

- **Secondary languages.** Given the increased diversity in our country, bilingualism is seen as a major plus-point by organizations. List this only if you are fluent in a second language. This means you are able to converse and interpret for others on your team.

- **Professional membership,** such as your membership in your state's student nurses' association or a nursing association on your campus, which demonstrates that you have an interest in your future profession.

- **Other categories.** Here you can include professional development and training you've undertaken that may support your new role. This section can be separate or you can include it as part of your education with the heading EDUCATION/TRAINING AND DEVELOPMENT. If you have written articles, participated in a research study, or hold a certification, include this on your résumé. Also, if you have served in the military, be sure to list that information as well (under the heading MILITARY SERVICE).

Watch out: While including all of the aforementioned information is crucial, DO NOT

- include salary requirements/history (unless requested)

- write the word "résumé" at the top of the page

- include a "references available upon request" line (you will have a separate page for this)

- exaggerate or misrepresent your experience

- use abbreviations

- use "I" statements

- list reasons for leaving a job

- include religious or political group affiliations

- attach a photograph or include a physical description of yourself

One page or two?

There is a long-standing debate on the appropriate length of a résumé. Contrary to popular belief, a one-page résumé is not always the best. If you decide on a two-page résumé be sure that you do not include unnecessary or trivial information. Think in terms of relevance, not the number of pages. If you do end up with a second page, be sure to list your contact information on that page, in case it becomes detached from the rest of the document. You could use the "header and footer" tool for this.

References page

The best way to handle the required reference and recommendation list is to put it on a separate page. Be sure to include your contact information on this page as well. Figure 1.2 provides an example of a reference sheet.

Figure 1.2: Reference sheet

Florence Nightingale
975 Warweary Way
Northmeadow, IL 60610
(403) 555-8732

REFERENCES

Business

Robert Newbold, Nurse Manager
General Hospital
1000 Brandyway Avenue
Willow, IL 60510
(403) 555-6913
RNewbold@willowhospital.org

Personal

Sally Ockajik, Registered Nurse
41 Susset Terrace
Willow, IL 60511
(403) 555-7531
sockajik@willowhospital.org

Wynette Mack,
Patient Care Associate
16 Pequabuck Street
Fairfield, IL
(403) 555-2351
wmack123@global.net

Academic

Nicole Ianacone,
Assistant Professor
Willow Community College
555 Batterson Avenue
Willow, IL 60511
(403) 555-1234
NIanacone@willow.comm.edu

Joanne DiValentino,
Assistant Professor
Willow Community College
555 Batterson Avenue
Willow, IL 60511
(403) 555-1235
JDiValentino@willow.comm.edu

Leslie Larkin, Associate Professor
Willow Community College
555 Batterson Avenue
Willow, IL 60511
(403) 555-1236
LLarkin@willow.comm.edu

Power Words

Include power words when you write your résumé and your cover letter. Also, keep a dictionary or thesaurus handy to help you find the right synonym.

Figure 1.3: Power words

✳ Achieved	✳ Focused	✳ Proposed
✳ Adapted	✳ Generated	✳ Recommended
✳ Analyzed	✳ Implemented	✳ Reduced
✳ Assisted	✳ Improved	✳ Reinforced
✳ Built	✳ Increased	✳ Researched
✳ Collected	✳ Initiated	✳ Revised
✳ Compiled	✳ Introduced	✳ Saved
✳ Conducted	✳ Maintained	✳ Solved
✳ Coordinated	✳ Managed	✳ Spearheaded
✳ Created	✳ Monitored	✳ Streamlined
✳ Decreased	✳ Organized	✳ Strengthened
✳ Delegated	✳ Participated	✳ Supported
✳ Demonstrated	✳ Performed	✳ Taught
✳ Drafted	✳ Planned	✳ Updated
✳ Established	✳ Prepared	
✳ Expanded	✳ Produced	

Figure 1.4: Model résumé

Carol Anne Burke
14 Covey Drive
Alabaster, MA 01234
Home: (213) 555-3694   Cell: (213) 555-7812
caburke@farscape.net

Desired position: Staff nurse

EMPLOYMENT
Patient Care Associate
Huntington Hospital
Huntington, MA
May 2004 – June 2006
Responsibilities and duties: Assisting the nurse in the care of medical-surgical patients.
Specialized skills: Phlebotomy, ECG, and minor respiratory therapy interventions.
Accomplishments and achievements: Employee of the month, September 2005.
Numerous patient satisfaction surveys that include my name for providing quality care
during the patient's hospitalization.

EDUCATION
Huntington Community College
Huntington, MA
Associate Degree in Nursing, 2006
Course Work: Medical-surgical: Huntington Hospital, Units F and G
Obstetrics: Women's Hospital, Boston, Unit 5
Pediatrics: Children's Hospital, Boston, Unit 9
Behavioral health: Long Lane Academy, Ashford, MA
Achievements, Awards/Scholarships: Dean's List for all semesters, Massachusetts
Nurses' Association Student Nurses' Foundation financial scholarship
Certifications: CPR, 2005

PROFESSIONAL MEMBERSHIPS
National Student Nurses' Association, 2004–2006
Student Nurses' Association, Huntington chapter – served as secretary

COMMUNITY SERVICE AND VOLUNTEER ACTIVITIES
Christ the King Catholic Church
Ashford, MA
Volunteer CCD teacher, 1999-2004

Habitat for Humanity
Boston, MA
Volunteer, 2000

Electronic résumé tips

In this age of technology, you may see an advertisement for a job that requires you to submit your résumé electronically. Using your MS Word or Word Perfect format may not work well as an electronic submission. You should save your document as a rich text format (RTF) file to ensure it looks like it should on the receiving end. You can either cut and paste it into the online job application form or send it as an attachment. Once you have written your text version, e-mail it to yourself or a friend to see how it looks before posting it.

Tip: Guidelines for submitting an electronic résumé

- Left-justify the entire document.

- Avoid fancy fonts or characters. Use Arial or Helvetica font in 12-point type size. Check with the job ad—they may prefer 10-point.

- Avoid tabs and hard returns. They do not translate well in the electronic format.

- Avoid italics, script, underlining, boldface, underscoring, and bullets. Use an asterisk or dash instead of bullets. Use capital letters for emphasis.

- Avoid using horizontal or vertical lines.

- Avoid faxed copies, as they may become fuzzy on the receiving end. If it is really necessary for the employer to get your résumé quickly, send it overnight express.

Cover letters

Once you have completed your research on the organization in which you are interested, you can sit down and write a custom cover letter. You did this research to develop a better understanding of the organization's mission, goals, and how well you will fit in. Keeping this in mind, your cover letter should demonstrate your interpretation of the organization's mission, how/why you feel you would be a good fit with the institution, and the skills and experience you offer. Do not repeat too much information that is already on your résumé, as this would just be wasting space. Just use key skills that are applicable to the job for which you are applying, if you feel it is necessary.

Don't forget: Cover letter rules

- Always send a cover letter with your résumé.

- Always address the letter to the appropriate individual. If you do not know his/her name and title, call the organization and ask.

- Always be clear and concise.

- Always limit the cover letter to three or four paragraphs.

- Always type your cover letter.

- Always use the same paper that you used for your résumé.

- Always proofread your cover letter very closely. (Then have someone else read it.)

- Always include the exact title of the position you are seeking.

- Always remember that the cover letter should indicate why you want to work for the organization. It should answer the question, "Why should I interview this nurse?"

- Always include a sample of what you know about the organization (based on the research you did). For example, you may want to cite the organization's impressive quality and clinical outcomes, their achievement of Magnet status, or their standing with patient or employee satisfaction scores.

Figure 1.5: Model cover letter

14 Covey Drive
Alabaster, MA 01234
Home: (213) 555-3694
Cell: (213) 555-7812
caburke@farscape.net

Mr. Herman Heinz
Human Resources Manager
Huntington Hospital
100 Grand Street
Huntington, MA 01235
March 12, 2006

Dear Mr. Heinz:

[Paragraph one: Explain why you are interested in the organization. Include any applicable, specific information concerning the organization, such as recently achieving JCAHO recertification.]

I am seeking a staff nurse position in your hospital. I believe that you will find my clinical background and experience aptly fit the criteria for the position openings on the medical-surgical unit. As I have had many of my clinical rotations at your hospital and have also served as a patient care associate at Huntington, I am very familiar with the organization and would love the opportunity to serve as a full-time staff member.

[Paragraph two: Briefly describe your clinical qualifications and accomplishments at school or work. Tie them into the job you are seeking.]

Currently, I am completing my senior rotation at Huntington Community College and ex-pect to graduate this May. Throughout nursing school, I have demonstrated the ambition to succeed and the ability to balance school work with part-time employment. As a PCA, I have received employee service awards due to my commitment to teamwork and patient satisfaction.

[Paragraph three: Take the initiative and ask for an interview. Provide possible dates and times you are available. Always include a thank you for the HR manager's time and consideration.]

Please let me know if you need any further information. I can provide references upon request. I am available on any Thursday and look forward to meeting with you to discuss employment options at your facility. Thank you for your time and consideration.

Sincerely,
(Handwritten signature)
Carol Anne Burke

Thank you letters

Writing a thank you letter is part of job-search etiquette. It can be brief, but should reflect what happened during the interview and your continued interest in the position. If you forgot to mention something important about yourself, this is a good opportunity for you to include it. You should send a thank you letter within a day of the interview. A letter needs to go to any-one with whom you have had a formal interview—the human resources manager, the nurse manager, and any staff member. Be sure to get the names of any staff members who were in the interview room before you leave the unit. Figure 1.6 is an example of a thank you letter to the nurse manager.

Figure 1.6: Model thank you letter

Florence Nightingale
975 Warweary Way
Northmeadow, IL 60610
(403) 555-8732

July 12, 2006

Nancy Brodey, Nurse Manager
Unit N12
Willow Hospital
Willow, IL 60510

Dear Ms. Brodey:

Please accept this letter as a thank you for taking time out of your busy day on Tuesday. It was a pleasure meeting you and your staff. I was most impressed by the high professional standards that your staff demonstrated. They shared their unit accomplishments with me and made me want to become a contributing member of your team.

I am certain that my willingness to continue to learn and grow in the role of new graduate would be an asset to your team. Your commitment to patient safety and meeting quality goals is admirable, and I would appreciate the opportunity to be part of this work.

Once again, thank you for your consideration and I look forward to hearing from you.

Sincerely,

[Handwritten signature]
Florence Nightingale

Figure 1.7: The ABCs of getting a job

A = Attitude	Make sure you have a positive one.
B = Benefits	Look at the information carefully, compare each potential employer, and call human resources with any questions.
C = Competencies	Always be honest. No one expects you to be an expert. You can talk about your current competencies and talk about which ones you still want to learn.
D = Directions	Get them. Be sure you know where you are going so that you are not late for the interview.
E = Eye Contact	Be sure of yourself and make direct eye contact during the interview.
F = Follow up	After every meeting/interview.
G = Goals	Set realistic goals and be prepared to talk about them if asked.
H = Handshake	Make it firm but not overpowering.
I = Interview	Remember it only takes one to get you through the door and into the right job.
J = Join	Joining organizations will show your commitment to the profession. Remember to list your affiliations on your resume.
K = Knowledge	Do your research and know the organization you are interested in.
L = Location	Decide where is best for you. Can you afford to relocate?
M = Money	Get paid what you are worth. Search nursing journals and the internet for the salary ranges for your region and level.
N = Network	Get to know as many people in the field as you can. This can be crucial when it comes to finding your dream job.
O = Organization	Make sure your materials are organized, as well as your appearance. Have extra copies of your resume on hand during your interview—it shows you are put together and prepared (especially if someone needs a copy).
P = Practice	Practice, practice, practice your interviewing skills.
Q = Questions	Be prepared to ask questions of your potential manager.
R = Résumé	It's you—on paper.
S = SOAR	S = situation, O = obstacles, A = action, and R = results. Be prepared to give one example. See next page for more information.
T = Thank you	Thank everyone who helped you before, during, and after the interview. Include those you asked for references and letters of recommendation.
U = Understand	Get to know and understand yourself so that you are self-assured during the interview.
V = Voice	Speak clearly and do not use "um" and "uh."
W = Writing	Your documents must be error-free and clean.
X = eXtra time	Take a few minutes to double and triple check all of your work. If the final decision for a position comes down to you and another candidate, that one misspelled word on your résumé may be the reason you lose out.
Y = Yahoo!	Be sure and take time to celebrate your success in graduating from nursing school, getting the job you wanted, and achieving your goals.
Z = Zero in	Keep your eye on the prize! When you focus on your goals, success comes naturally.

Preparing for the interview

The interview begins from the moment you enter the building. Be polite and appreciative with everyone you meet. A simple "thank you" will go a long way.

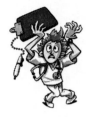

Don't panic: *SOAR*

If you are the type of person who does not like to talk about themselves, you need to read this! You have skills and accomplishments. The interviewer will almost always ask you to talk about an accomplishment or something of which you are proud. Look at the achievements and successes that have helped you define your skills and traits. Those are the important qualities for which a potential employer is looking.

The following exercise, called SOAR, will help you identify your skills so that you will be able to communicate them at the interview. Use the exercise to get ready for your interviews.

Situation: Describe a situation from your clinical or work experience.

Obstacles: Describe the obstacles you faced.

Actions: List the actions you took.

Results: Describe the results you helped obtain and the benefits to your employer/classmates/patient.

Try to think of three or more SOAR examples and incorporate them into your preparation and practice interview. The following is an example:

Situation: Decreasing patient falls on Unit 5.

Obstacles: Not enough patient safety equipment on the unit/not all PCAs committed to the Quality Improvement (QI) project of reducing falls on the unit.

Action: Met with my nurse manager and discussed my suggestions of doing an inventory of the existing patient safety equipment. Sent broken equipment to maintenance. Gave the results to the nurse manager to order more equipment and started PCA walking rounds at the change of shift.

Results: Patient falls dropped by 50%.

Interviewing skills

First, you need to dress for success. You cannot expect to land the job of your dreams looking like a college student. Think of this job interview as a business exchange. You are selling yourself and they are looking to buy the best product on the market. So, you need to spend some time and money on yourself. Consider this an excuse to go and buy that new suit or professional-looking outfit. The return on this investment will be well worth it. Look groomed, neat, and "put together." If you look as if you are successful, you will be successful.

Second, if you are not good at interviewing or have never had a job interview before now, you will need to practice, practice, practice. Use your colleagues or a faculty member for mock interviews. Honing your interviewing skills will help you land the job you really want. Remember, the first five minutes of every interview are the most critical. The decision to hire is made with first impressions.

Figure 1.8 lists some examples of interview questions and why they are used.

Figure 1.8: Sample interview questions and rationales

Question	Rationale
Tell me about yourself.	Getting to know you
What will you bring to this position?	Self-awareness skills
What would you consider to be your best and worst traits?	Identifies your strengths and weaknesses
Describe a clinical assignment that did not turn out the way you planned. What did you do?	Problem-solving skills
What did you learn from that assignment?	Ability to learn from mistakes
Tell me what interests you about this position.	Interest
Describe a situation in which you had to work with someone you did not like.	Ability to work on a team
Describe how you would deal with an upset patient or family member.	Customer-focused skills
For what type of personality do you do your best work?	Working with management
Describe a situation in which you had to learn a lot in a short period of time. How did you manage this and what was the outcome?	Learning and initiative skills
Where do you predict nursing is going in the future?	Knowledge of the profession
Would you report yourself if you made a mistake?	Integrity
What do you do to alleviate stress?	Stress management skills
How well did you manage your assignments as a student nurse?	Organization skills
I am going to give you an assignment of the following three patients. How would you manage their care? Who would you go see first?	Prioritization skills
How would you handle a situation where someone for whom you were responsible made a serious mistake?	People skills Performance management skills
Where do you see yourself in five years?	Ambition

Asking the right questions

Think of the interview process as a two-way conversation. It is important for you to ask questions to ensure that you are picking the right organization, and that it matches your personality, philosophy, and pay needs. Asking the right questions will get you the information you need to match your qualifications to the job. You will be able to evaluate the position and make a sound decision as to whether it is the right job for you.

Think in terms of question categories, such as

- Responsibilities of the position

- Resources available to meet the responsibilities (e.g., staffing, supplies, educational support such as orientation programs and continuing education)

- Performance measurements and timeframes

- Organization and unit culture

Sample questions to ask human resources and the nurse manager

When you start your interview process you will first have to meet with the nurse recruiter or human resources manager. They will go over the generalities of the organization, the benefits, and information about the position for which you are interviewing. They will then ask you if you have any questions for them. You should be prepared to ask insightful questions. This is your chance to find out if this is the right job for you.

 Ask: In addition to the title of the position, the salary range, the length of the orientation program, and the anticipated shift hours, you can ask

- How long have you been with the organization?

- Why do you enjoy working for this organization?

- How would you describe the philosophy of the organization?

- In your opinion, what is the most important contribution that this organization expects from its employees?

- What is the next step in the interview process?

In order to understand the level of competition for the position, what the position really entails, and what the style of the management team is, you could ask

- How do my skills compare with those candidates you have interviewed?

- What advice would you give to a new graduate?

- Can I have a written job description?

- Can you talk about the organization's commitment to equal opportunity and diversity?

- Is the executive team visible to the employee?

- What is the management style in the department of nursing?

When you meet with your prospective nurse manager, you want to demonstrate that you are prepared and should ask

- How long have you been with the organization?

- What attracted you to this organization?

- How would you describe your management style?

- How would you describe the level of teamwork on the unit?

- What specific skills from the new graduate would make your life and the team's life easier? What are some of the skills and abilities you see as necessary for a new graduate to succeed on this unit?

- How long is your orientation program? What are the details of the program? Do orientees receive feedback from their preceptors and staff? If so, how often?

- What are some of the challenges that I might encounter if I take this position?

- Can you give me an idea of the typical day and workload of this position?

- What is the availability of the physician after hours?

- What are the three most important goals for the unit?

- What do you see as the most important areas for improvement? Is there a way that the staff can help?

- Is it possible to meet with some of the staff nurses?

- How soon are you looking to fill this position?

Keeping track of it all

As your job search will most likely happen during the school year, you will surely be busy during this time. You will need a way to keep track of all of your submitted applications, cover letters and résumés, as well as any telephone calls made and received, and any follow-up and thank you letters sent. Figure 1.9 provides a handy checklist for you to use.

Figure 1.9: Job-search checklist

Organization address/phone	Date application/ résumé sent	Interview date/time	Thank-you letter sent after interview (date)	Job offer received (date)	Notes

Professional courtesy

After completing your interviews, you will likely be contacted by a prospective employer. **If you are expecting more than one offer, that's okay. But it is not okay to say yes to all offers and then decide which one is best.**

Watch out: A Vice President for Nursing once told me that when a new graduate accepts a position with their facility but then goes to another facility, that new graduate is remembered and will not have another chance at her facility.

The professional way to handle multiple offers is to be honest and ask for more time to consider the offer. If Hospital A calls and makes you an offer, but you really prefer Hospital B, then thank them for the offer and ask if you can get back to them in 7–10 days. That way, you are still showing interest but also letting them know that you need more time to decide. Next, call Hospital B and ask them when they are planning to make a decision.

It is always okay to ask for time to consider any offer. Never say yes to an offer at the time of the offer. Tell the employer you'd like to call them back, and also tell them when you will call them back with your decision. Everyone should "sleep on" their big decisions.

References

Greiner, A., and A. Hendrich. 2006. Advancing Knowledge through Collaboration: Putting nurses in the driver's seat. *Reflections on Nursing Leadership.* 2nd quarter. *www.nursingsociety.org/RNL/Current/feature7.html.*

Provenzano, S. 2000. *Top Secret Executive Résumés.* Franklin Lake, NJ: The Career Press, Inc.

Upenieks, V. 2002. Assessing Differences in Job Satisfaction of Nurses in Magnet and Non-Magnet Hospitals. *Journal of Nursing Administration* 32(11): 564-576.

Thibeault, S. 2006. *Stressed Out About Nursing School.* 2nd edition. Marblehead, MA: HCPro, Inc.

Zerwekh, J., and J. Claborn. 2006. *Nursing Today: Transition and Trends.* 5th edition. St. Louis, MO: Saunders Elsevier.

Chapter 2

Today's demands on the nursing graduate

The nursing shortage: The facts

As a rising member of the nursing profession, you are acutely aware of the nursing shortage. You've read the studies and understand there is a growing gap between nurse supply and demand. You may even know that the U.S. Bureau of Labor Statistics estimates that there will be a shortfall of more than one million nurses by 2012. But do you know *why* the shortage is surging?

Fact: There are three elements that can explain the current nursing shortage in the United States today: 1) there is a demographic "perfect storm" occurring, 2) there are spiraling healthcare costs, and 3) there is an inability of the nursing education system to meet the demand for education. In fact, there is a nursing faculty shortage, which is also contributing to the third element.

A demographic "perfect storm"

This first element should not surprise you. The Baby Boomer generation—those born between 1946 and 1964—is getting older. As they age, Baby Boomers will develop chronic illnesses, which will put a strain on healthcare resources and dollars. There will also be many more aging Americans who naturally develop chronic conditions because we are living longer.

Within the Baby Boomer generation is also the largest population of nurses, many of whom are approaching retirement. According to statistics, most

Baby Boomers will reach retirement age by 2020 (O'Neil 2006). But as these nurses leave the profession, there are not nearly enough people to replace them—enrollments in nursing schools would have to increase at least 40% to meet the needs of the retirement-aged workforce.

Spiraling healthcare costs

As healthcare costs, which represent a whopping 16% of the total gross domestic product (GDP), continue to trend upward, hospitals are being forced to redistribute their resources (O'Neil 2006). The resources that nurses need to give care have decreased, even as the acuity level of the patients has increased. Patient admissions are down as well as the length of stay, even though patients today have much more complex problems than in the past. As Edward O'Neil, MPA, PhD, FAAN, director of the Center for Health Professions at the University of California at San Francisco said, "the hospital has become a pressure cooker environment" (O'Neil 2006).

The struggling nursing education system

There was a time when nursing schools had declining enrollments. But that has changed and the demand for nursing education has rebounded. Nursing schools are now faced with turning away potential applicants who desperately want to become nurses. Why are they being turned away? Just as there is a nursing shortage, there is also a shortage of nurse educators, classroom space, clinical preceptors, money, and clinical sites.

The future of the shortage: How it affects you

The nursing shortage is not only a present problem, but one that will worsen in time. In the past when there was a nursing shortage, the solution was simply to increase the supply. Education was made more accessible, nursing salaries were increased due to the demand, and the problem was solved in less than five years. But today's shortage is more complex than in the past— according to nurse researcher Peter Buerhaus, PhD, RN, FAAN, more than 75% of RNs believe the nursing shortage presents a major problem for the quality of their work life, the quality of patient care, and the amount of time they can spend with their patients. Almost all the nurses Buerhaus surveyed saw the nursing shortage in the future contributing to even more stress on nurses, lowered patient quality, and one of the major causes of nurses leaving their profession (Buerhaus et al. 2005).

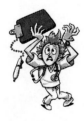

Don't panic: As a new nurse, you need to know the facts about the nursing shortage so that you can understand the reality of what nurses are facing today. It is not all that grim. In fact, administrators, legislators, and nursing schools have all been working hard on developing tactics to combat the problem.

Healthcare organizations have been using many different strategies to face the shortage. O'Neil has broken down these responses into four different categories: the scramble response, the improve response, the reinvent response, and the start-over response (O'Neil 2006). You may see some of these in your own job.

The scramble response

These are the simple and short-term solutions to the problem. Organizations see the nurse as a commodity and think the solution is to just increase the number of nurses—you may see healthcare organizations use a public-relations campaign as a recruitment tool to accomplish this. Some organizations may also provide educational scholarships (or tuition reimbursement), use sign-on bonuses, use travel or foreign nurses, or entice nurses with loan-forgiveness programs. Other short-term strategies may include raising salaries, retention or referral bonuses, implementing flexible self-schedule systems, and offering a broader range of shift types (O'Neil 2006). Remember that these have been used in the past and are certainly only a band-aid to the nursing shortage. Only you can decide if they work for you.

The improve response

This response focuses on the nurse as a customer and seeks to improve the nursing profession as a whole, instead of just implementing quick fixes. To do this, organizations are providing educational opportunities for nurses, increasing the number of nurse-driven quality-improvement initiatives, and seeking to achieve ANCC Magnet Recognition Program® designation. In an effort to improve the transition of new graduates, there have also been efforts to increase the number and efficiency of mentoring and nurse residency programs.

Nursing schools are working to improve by increasing the number of nursing faculty, recruiting underrepresented students to improve nursing diversity, and changing their curriculum to better integrate nursing practice into nursing education (O'Neil 2006).

The reinvent response

This response uses long-term strategies. Here, nurses are seen as a valued asset to the organization—i.e., nursing leadership recognizes that nurses play a crucial role in helping the organization achieve its goals of patient satisfaction, patient safety, and efficient use of resources. Now that's what you call empowerment!

Under this mentality, nurses also have an opportunity to *take the lead* in making their organization patient-friendly, safe, and highly regarded by patients and staff alike. In any organization, nurses have the power to do this and so much more—it is simply a matter of believing in ourselves and realizing our full potential.

The start-over response

This category of solutions may be considered "forward thinking," meaning it takes into consideration the next 15 to 20 years, when the nursing shortage will be at a critical level. As organizations are recognizing that there are certain things changing in healthcare (e.g., technology and the workforce), they are seeking to start over with new assumptions. They may begin looking at reorganizing nurses' practices around the treatment of the chronically ill in the home and community setting, or they may start examining what the technology will be in the future and how to use it.

Under this response, smart hospital and nursing administrations will look at the nursing shortage as a job development opportunity and not a workforce problem. They will understand that we cannot simply "patch" the problem of the growing nursing shortage, but instead must look for creative ways to attract and retain the nursing workforce of both today and tomorrow.

Figure 2.1: Where is my organization?

Short-term strategies	Long-term strategies
Temporary staff Per diem, travel nurses, float pool, internal staffing agency, online shift auction	*Nurse education* New schools, flexible hours for those attending school, nurse extern programs, tuition reimbursement, orientation programs (lengthening, redesigning), partnerships with nursing schools
Salary and financial benefits Competitive salaries; wage increases; sign-on, retention and/or referral bonuses	*Nurses' work environment* Positive changes in work environment, increased staffing levels, changing roles and responsibilities, physical changes to nurses' station
Flexible schedules Broader range of shift types; self-scheduling, two-hour "parent shifts"	*Strategic planning* Research into the future of the nursing shortage; development of practical, long-term solutions (e.g., succession planning, technological improvements)

Source: May, J. et al. 2006. Hospitals' Responses to Nursing Staffing Shortages. Health Affairs *25(4): w316-w323.* http://content.healthaffairs.org/cgi/content/abstract/hlthaff.25.w316.

30

What can I do?

It is time to think out of the box, and you can be part of it. Permanent solutions need to developed to combat this growing problem. Everyone, especially nurses, should be looking at solutions and talking about what is possible versus what is impossible.

Tip: Here are some actions that the healthcare community—of which you are a part—can take:

- Create new models of care that have the nurse at the center of safe, high-quality patient care

- Dedicate more money to looking at healthcare outcomes and patient satisfaction

- Reinvent nursing education to address the future generation of nurses

- Change the work environment for nurses so that healthcare facilities are safer places for nurses to work

Help is coming

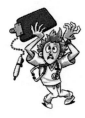

Don't panic: We know that if hospitals give nurses a say in how they care for patients, solutions for this nursing shortage will surface. Nurses are likely to make recommendations that will deliver safer, more effective care—leaving them and their patients feeling more satisfied.

There is currently a national study being conducted on nurses' professional habits called Transforming Care at the Bedside (TCAB). It is an initiative of the Robert Wood Johnson Foundation and the Institute for Healthcare Improvement designed to improve the quality and safety of patient care and increase the retention of experienced nurses. This study is looking at the amount of time nurses spend at the nurses' station and walking during their shift. The goal is to find ways to improve the nurses' work environment. By doing this, researchers hope that there will be an improvement in efficiency and a reduction in medical errors. The study will help hospitals make adjustments to the workplace in terms of nursing schedules and floor plans, which will improve not only nurses' efficiency, but patient safety as well. In turn, the nursing environment will be made less stressful.

Other studies have also indicated that improvements are on the horizon. For example, a study published in the June 2006 issue of the journal *Health Affairs* reported that 88% of 32 hospitals in 12 nationally representative markets said they have made changes to the nursing work environment. Some of these changes included

- altering nurse staffing levels

- repositioning nursing roles and responsibilities

- making nursing units more accessible and nurse-friendly

- implementing quality-improvement efforts (May et al. 2006)

Stresses and challenges for the new graduate

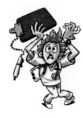

Don't panic: You are entering one of the most rewarding professions in the world. Nurses are highly respected and trusted by the public. Nurses touch lives in many ways and are remembered by patients and families for the care they provide. Along with the job title, however, come a number of stressors—stressors that make the job of nursing one of the most challenging of all fields. With that in mind, there are realities that you need to know *from the beginning* so that you are prepared and can manage the stresses that come with this noble profession.

Watch out: You probably already know some of the factors that you will face on the nursing unit:

- Rapid turnover of nursing staff or lack of adequate nursing staff

- Increasing patient acuity

- Shorter stays in the hospital

- An aging workforce

Ask: In addition to the challenges of the work environment, you will be facing the challenge of being a new graduate. How will you cope with the challenges of this new role? How will you handle some of the stressors of the work environment, such as fulfilling the high job demands of nursing, coping with a lack of support from your peers, floating to other nursing units, and struggling with work overload due to poor prioritization and time management? **You need to face these questions and learn how to manage them in this critical first year—if you don't, the result will be that you will see nursing as a stressful and less-satisfying career than you expected.**

Let's begin by tackling the realities you will face, as studies have shown that clinical practice is often very stressful for new graduates.

Concerns exercise: What are you most worried about?

Put the following list of concerns in order from 1–8, with 1 being the concern you think will cause you most stress, and 8 being the concern that will cause you the least.

_____ Inconsistent preceptor

_____ Encountering new situations, surroundings, and procedures

_____ Not feeling confident and competent

_____ Staff nurses who are unwilling to help

_____ Making mistakes because of increased workload and responsibilities

_____ Encounters with unhappy nurses and other personnel

_____ Getting to know the staff

_____ Short staffing (Oermann and Garvin 2002)

Now compare your responses to the most common ranking provided by new graduates who participated in a study on this topic—the list can be found at the end of this chapter (Oermann and Garvin 2002).

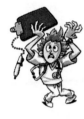

Don't panic: You'll see you are not alone. New graduates say that they have moderate levels of stress even in their orientation period because of their lack of clinical experience and organizational skills (Oermann and Garvin 2002). Later in this book, we'll discuss moving from novice to expert. You cannot expect to be an expert nurse within the first year of nursing practice—you will be functioning at the advanced-beginner level. Do not put unrealistic expectations on yourself and do not let anyone else do it either. In order to deal effectively with the stress of the job, you must first ask yourself "What is the cause of my stress?" It may be

- assuming increasing responsibility

- not feeling confident and competent

- making mistakes because of an increased workload and responsibilities

- short staffing

- being tired

- informing patients and families of negative findings

- working with terminally ill and dependent patients

- discharging patients too soon

- staff nurses who are unwilling to help you (Oermann and Garvin 2002)

Clearly, you see that you are going to encounter "role stress." Role stress happens when there is a difference between what you perceive the role of the nurse to be and what is actually happening in the role. You may become upset because there is a wide gap between what the role expectation is and what can actually be accomplished. Burnout then occurs, as a result of work overload, lack of social support, and role stress. Signs and symptoms of burnout include absenteeism, lack of work satisfaction, feelings of inadequacy, irritability, depression, somatic problems, and sleep disorders (Chang and Hancock 2003). You will see this in other nurses and hopefully recognize it in yourself before it is too late.

Strategies to reduce role stress

There are a number of strategies you can use to control your stress—strategies you may even want to share with your fellow nurses and nursing administration:

1. Understand yourself so that you can build relationships with your colleagues.

2. Never be afraid to ask questions. It is okay to let people know that you do not have the answer. Nursing is a lifelong learning profession.

3. Know your limitations. Do not be afraid to express them in a professional manner when asked to do something that makes you feel uncomfortable.

4. Be a sponge and soak up as much as you can—watch and listen and you will learn so much more than what you learned in school.

5. Find a personal mentor and ask him/her to be your support person for at least the first year. You will need to talk to someone about your good and bad days in nursing.

6. Always have integrity—with it, you will gain the trust and respect of everyone with whom you come in contact.

7. Do it right the first time, even if you think there is no time. Chances are, you won't have time to do it over.

8. Develop good organization skills. Do not save things for later—there may not be a later.

9. Do not complain about something (or someone) unless you have a solution. No one likes a complainer.

10. Listen to your patients; they know their bodies better than you do.

Fitting into the work environment

> *People acting together as a group can accomplish things which no individual acting alone could ever bring about.*
> –Franklin Roosevelt

As a new graduate you will have to learn to work with many different personalities and work "cultures." To do this successfully, you must understand yourself and how you work so that you can fit into the team with which you are working.

Socialization or fitting in on your unit is as important as increasing your nursing skills. If you do not work at trying to be part of the team, your experience at work may not be a happy one and you may run the risk of becoming one of the statistics of new-grad turnover.

Tip: The following are some tips on fitting in:

- Take your breaks off the unit and with your teammates. Do not isolate yourself in the breakroom.

- Take the first step and make every effort to get to know your coworkers. Ask them about themselves, their family, their grandchildren, pets, outside hobbies, etc. Listen to what they have to say.

- Avoid getting involved in any workplace gossip or issues, which can lead to conflict and interpersonal tension. This just adds to an already stressful work environment.

- If there is a retirement or holiday party, join in. Or better yet, since you are the newest member of the team, offer to work for one of the more senior members. That will certainly win you some points.

- Every once in awhile bring food to the breakroom. It doesn't have to be home made—everyone likes a good coffee cake or some bagels with their coffee.

Healthcare today is complex and demanding. The patients we care for are sicker and demand more of our energy. Years ago we relied on a nursing model called team nursing. It was a functional team on which everyone had a designated role and worked together to get the job done. Then, we transitioned to the patient-centered nursing care model. At first, both the nursing staff and patients liked this model, but as the healthcare system changed, nurses were asked to do more with less and with fewer professional colleagues. We have not fully recovered from this change and that is why working as a "team" has become so essential for our survival. It's also why you need to be sure that you work at fitting in.

Just think about all the different people on the unit. There are housekeeping staff, dietary staff, nurse extenders (patient care assistants), unit secretaries, physicians, physician assistants, nurses, technicians, and many others. How will you work with them? How will they work with you? To be an effective team member you need to understand your role on the team. You role may change with every new project, crisis, or nursing intervention. For a team to be considered a high-performing team, they must be willing to work together to achieve the best outcome. Sit back and try to figure out which of your coworkers fulfill the following roles. In a year or so, it will be your turn to decide which one you want to be.

- **Initiator:** spearheads actions and processes that promote team development

- **Model:** shapes behaviors that reflect expectations set for the team

- **Coach:** serves as a counselor, mentor, and tutor to help team members improve performance.

Even as a new graduate, you have a role on the team—you are a participant. Though you are learning, you can still prove to your team that you are a willing and able new member. In fact, you may see the situation differently than the rest of the team, and that new perspective may just be the key to solving the problem or accomplishing the outcome needed. So don't be afraid to roll up your sleeves and pitch in. And remember: there is no "I" in team.

 Fact: Here are some benefits to being a part of a team:

- Improved performance

- Increased motivation

- Better ability to respond quickly to changes

- Shared commitment to goals

- Greater creativity and problem-solving

- Improved communication

Bridging the generation gap

Today's workforce has four different generations working together. Each has their own set of values, ideals, traits, and goals. These differences include communication styles, expectations, work ethic, comfort level with technology, perceptions of loyalty, and acceptance of change. If such differences are not understood by all involved, they can lead to a misunderstanding of each other and, ultimately, to conflict. As a new nurse, make it a priority to understand each generation—not only will it help you relate to others outside of your generation, but it will help them relate to you as well.

The Silent Generation: Born before 1945

This generation of nurses makes up about 10% of the workforce today. "Silents" have been described as unimaginative, unadventurous, cautious, and withdrawn—thus the name (Strauss and Howe 1991). Growing up, they were taught to rely on the tried and true way of doing things. They believe in dedication, commitment, loyalty and a hard day's work. They are respectful of authority, support administration, and work with discipline. Members of this generation prefer to work in large organizations that offer job security and other non-monetary benefits. They recognize that cutting-edge thinking and new technologies will help them stay on top of nursing.

Watch out: Do not stereotype this group. What they lack in technology expertise they make up for in their listening, conflict resolution, and problem-solving skills (Martin 2004). Consult these individuals for their experience with patient problems. They have seen it all.

Baby Boomers: Born between 1946 and 1964

This generation represents approximately 45% of today's workforce (Martin 2004). During their formative years, society encouraged them to think as individuals and express themselves creatively. Many Boomers feel that they have already paid their dues and put in the necessary effort to climb up the professional ladder. Now, however, they find themselves under new rules—rules where seniority is not always the deciding factor.

After watching the Gen Xers get hiring bonuses and plum schedules, they are now asking for the respect and recognition that they deserve due to their significant contributions. Go to these people when you need coaching and mentoring.

Generation X: Born between 1965 and 1980

This generation makes up about 30% of the workforce (Martin 2004). The first generation to recognize from the beginning that job security is a myth, Gen Xers want to learn useful skills and have a job that will promote their financial security, while still being able to enjoy their leisure time. They anger the Silents and Baby Boomers because of their "free agent" attitude. However, in the past 10 years this generation has proved itself valuable. They are creative contributors who have a drive to get things done in a smarter/faster/safer way. They are the ones who have changed the workplace for the better for all nurses.

Generation Y/Millennial Generation: Born between 1980 and 2006

About 15% of the workforce today consists of this generation—the generation you may very well be a part of it (Martin 2004). Born to the Baby Boomer generation, Gen Yers were encouraged to learn and express themselves. This resulted in high levels of self-confidence.

Gen Yers believe that education is the key to their success. They grew up with technology and accept diversity. This generation likes new challenges and opportunities. They are considered to be positive, assertive, civic, and moral individuals. With these traits, the Gen Yers have the potential to be the most productive workforce in history.

Generation Y nurses should use mentors to serve as experienced guides who can help them to succeed. Although they have the knowledge and skills that will make them competent, Gen Yers need to learn how to ask good questions—and listen carefully to those who have the experience (Martin 2004).

Figure 2.2: Generational characteristics

Generation	Core Values	Characteristics
Silent 1926-1945	Loyalty/Commitment Dedication Self-discipline Sacrifice Hard work Tradition Conformity Respect Adherence to rules	• Value hard work • Emphasize traditional mores • Value job security and loyalty to company • Listen to others • Place well-being of others before themselves • Value religion and patriotism
Baby Boomer 1946-1964	Hard work Individualism Optimism Self-will Teamwork Personal growth Education Dedication Personal gratification	• Place high value on their career and climbing the professional ladder • Dedicated to learning • Feel a sense of entitlement for the work they have done • Question the establishment/act rebellious • Use passive-aggressiveness to deal with conflict • Take risks and "dream big"
X 1965-1980	Change Independence/Self-reliance Education Culture/Thinking globally Work/Life balance Fun Success Informality Pragmatism	• See themselves as forward-thinkers and individualists • Interested in immediate, tangible needs • Embrace technology • Dislike stagnancy/Thrive on continual change and challenges • Have great respect for knowledge and learning • Criticized as being self-absorbed, cynical, and dismissive
Y/Millennial 1981-2006	Flexibility Optimism Family Insight/Thought Confidence Civic duty Achievement Diversity	• Have respect for parents and family • See future with optimism/positivism • Prefer to multitask • Value sensibility • Welcome guidance/Accept authority • Believe they will be successful/rich • Gravitate toward group activities • Think of themselves in a global context

Source: Ski, J. 2006. A Practical Guide to Managing the Multigenerational Workforce: Skills for Nurse Managers. Marblehead, MA: HCPro, Inc.

Words of wisdom: Remembering how we treat people

 Don't forget: Now that you understand where each generation is coming from, hopefully you see that we're not all that different from one another, and that our differences can actually strengthen our team. No matter what our age, our appearance, or our personality, we are all nurses, and we all must come together in the name of care.

The following are five lessons to help you think about the way we treat people.

Lesson #1: Understanding what's in a name

During my second month of college, our professor gave us a pop quiz. I was a conscientious student and had breezed through the questions until I reached the last one: "What is the first name of the woman who cleans the school?"

Surely, this was some kind of joke. I had seen the cleaning woman several times. She was tall, dark-haired, and in her 50s, but how would I know her name? I handed in my paper, leaving the last question blank. Just before class ended, one student asked if the last question would count toward our quiz grade.

"Absolutely," said the professor. "In your careers, you will meet many people. All are significant. They deserve your attention and care, even if all you do is smile and say 'hello.'"

I've never forgotten that lesson. And I also learned her name was Dorothy.

Lesson #2: Helping those in need

One night, at 11:30 p.m., an older African-American woman walked along an Alabama highway, trying to endure a lashing rainstorm. Her car had broken down and she desperately needed a ride. Soaking wet, she decided to flag down the next car. A young white man stopped to help her—an action generally unheard of in those conflict-filled 1960s. The man took her to safety, helped her get assistance, and put her into a taxicab. She seemed to be in a big hurry, but she took down his address and thanked him.

Several days went by and a knock came at the man's door. To his surprise, a giant color TV was delivered to his home. A special note was attached. It read: "Thank you so much for assisting me on the highway the other night. The rain drenched not only my clothes, but also my spirits. Then you came along. Because of you, I was able to make it to my dying husband's bedside just before he passed away. God bless you for helping me and unselfishly serving others. Sincerely, Mrs. Nat King Cole."

Lesson #3: Remembering those who serve

In the days when an ice cream sundae cost much less, a 10-year-old boy entered a coffee shop and sat at a table. A waitress put a glass of water in front of him. "How much is an ice cream sundae?" he asked.

"Fifty cents," replied the waitress. The little boy pulled his hand out of his pocket and studied the coins in it.

"Well, how much is a plain dish of ice cream?" he inquired.

By now, more people were waiting for a table and the waitress was growing inpatient. "Thirty-five cents," she brusquely replied.

The little boy again counted his coins. "I'll have the plain ice cream," he said.

The waitress brought the ice cream, put the bill on the table and walked away. The boy finished the ice cream, paid the cashier and left. When the waitress came back, she began to cry as she wiped down the table. There, placed neatly beside the empty dish, were two nickels and five pennies. You see, he couldn't have the sundae, because he had to have enough left to leave her a tip.

Lesson #4: Removing obstacles in our path

In ancient times, a king had a boulder placed on a roadway. Then, he hid himself and watched to see if anyone would remove the huge rock. Some of the king's wealthiest merchants and courtiers came by and simply walked around it. Many loudly blamed the king for not keeping the roads clear, but none did anything about getting the stone out of the way.

Then, a peasant came along carrying a load of vegetables. Upon approaching the boulder, the peasant laid down his burden and tried to move the stone to the side of the road. After much pushing and straining, he finally succeeded. After the peasant picked up his load of vegetables, he noticed a purse lying in the road where the boulder had been. The purse contained many gold coins and a note from the King indicating that the gold was for the person who removed the boulder from the roadway. The peasant learned what many of us never understand—every obstacle presents an opportunity to improve our condition.

Lesson #5: Giving when it counts

Many years ago, when I worked as a volunteer at a hospital, I got to know a little girl named Liz who was suffering from a rare and serious disease. Her only chance of recovery appeared to be a blood transfusion from her five-year old brother, who had miraculously survived the same disease and had developed the antibodies needed to combat the illness. The doctor explained the situation to her brother, and asked the little boy if he would be willing to give his blood to his sister. I saw him hesitate for only a moment before taking a deep breath and saying, "Yes, I'll do it if it will save her."

As the transfusion progressed, he lay in bed next to his sister and smiled, as we all did, seeing the color return to her cheeks. Then his face grew pale and his smile faded. He looked up at the doctor and asked in a trembling voice, "Will I start to die right away?"

Being so young, the little boy had misunderstood the doctor; he thought he was going to have to give his sister all of his blood in order to save her.

Concerns exercise: Answers

Most frequently reported stressors new graduates face (1 being the concern that causes the most stress among the new graduates surveyed, 8 being the concern that causes the least):

1. Not feeling confident and competent
2. Making mistakes because of increased workload and responsibilities
3. Encountering new situations, surroundings, and procedures
4. Inconsistent preceptors
5. Getting to know the staff
6. Encounters with unhappy nurses and other personnel
7. Short staffing
8. Staff nurses who are unwilling to help (Oermann and Garvin 2002)

References

Buerhaus, P., et al. 2005. Part One: Is the shortage of hospital registered nurses getting better or worse? Findings from two recent national surveys of RNs. *Nursing Economic$* 23: 61–71, 96.

Chang, E., and K. Hancock. 2003. Role Stress and Role Ambiguity in New Nursing Graduates in Australia. *Nursing and Health Sciences* 5: 155–163.

Hart, S. 2006. Generational Diversity: Impact on Recruitment and Retention of Registered Nurses. *Journal of Nursing Administration* 36(1): 10–12.

Hill, K. 2004. Defy the decades with multigenerational teams. *Nursing Management* 5(1): 32–35.

Hu, J. et al. 2004. Managing the Multigenerational Nursing Team. *The Healthcare Manager* 23(4): 334–340.

Johnson, S., and M. Romanello. 2005. Generational Diversity Teaching and Learning Approaches. *Nurse Educator* 30(5): 212–216.

Martin, C. 2004. Bridging the Generation Gap(s). *Nursing 2004* 34(12): 62–63.

May, J. et al. 2006. Hospitals' Responses to Nursing Staffing Shortages. *Health Affairs* 25(4): w316–w323. *http://content.healthaffairs.org/cgi/content/abstract/hlthaff.25.w316.*

Oermann, M., and M. Garvin. 2002. Stresses and challenges for new graduates in hospitals. *Nurse Education Today* 22(3): 225–230.

O'Neil, E. 2006. Part 1 and Part 2: The Nursing Shortage, By the Numbers. Robert Wood Johnson Foundation. *www.rwjf.org.*

Strauss, W., and N. Howe. 1991. *Generations: The History of America's Future.* New York: William Morrow.

Part Two

Starting your first job can be a scary experience. But knowing how to get the most from orientation and understanding your transition from student nurse to RN can help keep you from becoming overwhelmed.

Chapter 3

Orientation: One of the keys to a successful transition

Do your best every day, and your life will gradually expand into satisfying fullness.

–Alexander Graham Bell

The real learning begins

You made it through nursing school, you passed the NCLEX exam, you landed a job—what could be harder? Well, how about being let go to function on your own? Sounds scary, doesn't it?

 Fact: One of the greatest fears of a new graduate is the fear of leaving the security of their instructors and being left on their own (McMahon 2005). The stress that new nurses face arises from the gap between the knowledge learned in school and the application of that knowledge in nursing care. In reality, as a new graduate, you will lack an understanding of the concepts and standards of care for your patients. This is to be expected. You are still in the novice phase of your nursing career and should not expect to be proficient in your first year. The organization should expect you to have limited technological, problem solving, and organizational skills. While there may be an expectation from some people that you should be able to "hit the ground running," this is an unrealistic expectation and one you should not put on yourself. Consider yourself a nurse intern for the first year.

Enjoy your new grad experience as it won't be there again.
−2005 Graduate

Welcome to orientation

Orientation provides time for you to strengthen your nursing skills and work on your critical thinking abilities in a supportive environment. During the orientation period, you will work on your competencies, learn about the role of the nurse, figure out how to deal with the rigors of the work environment, and improve your organizational and prioritization skills. At the end of your orientation, you should be able to make safe decisions and carry out the normal standards of care for the unit assigned.

A good orientation program will

- offer a reassuring and warm welcome at the beginning of employment and treat new nurses humanely

- offer complete and precise training from the onset

- train supervisors and provide them with the tools to measure the continuing progress of professional competence

- offer constant support for new nurses

- evaluate the orientation program on a permanent basis (Lavoie-Tremblay et al. 2002)

The following figure illustrates a sample agenda for the first four weeks of orientation.

Figure 3.1: Sample week-to-week orientation schedule

SAINT FRANCIS HOSPITAL AND MEDICAL CENTER
DEPARTMENT OF PATIENT CARE SERVICES
Center for Clinical Excellence and Professional Development

Medical/Surgical Orientation Program
Entry-Level Registered Nurse—Medical/Surgical Units

Name: _____ **Employee ID#:** _____

Orientation Start Date: _____

Orientation End Date: _____

WEEK ONE: Date: _____

OBJECTIVE:
- To assist the entry level registered nurse in the development of his/her professional role within an acute care setting.
- To introduce the entry-level registered nurse to the Professional Nursing Practice Model and Patient Focused Care of Saint Francis Hospital and Medical Center.
- To introduce the new employee to the organizational policies, programs and resources of Saint Francis Care.

GOALS:

The orientee will complete	Date	Initials
1. Human Resource Orientation		
2. Patient Care Service Orientation		
3. 14 hours of Medical/Surgical Practicum		
4. IDX Training		
5. Math Calculation Test with an 80% score		

Figure 3.1: Sample week-to-week orientation schedule (cont.)

WEEK TWO: Date: _____

OBJECTIVE:
- To assist the entry-level registered nurse in the integration of professional and clinical competencies when caring for adults of all ages.
- To provide adequate time for unit and organization familiarization and socialization.

GOALS:

The orientee will	Date	Initials
1. Complete "Work Area Orientation Guide" (found in Orientation Packet) with staff RN		
2. Review Unit Structure Standards/ Population Types/Generic Structure Standards with Nurse Manager		
3. Review Resource Manuals on Unit		
4. Complete Medical/Surgical Practicum		
5. Shadow and assist RN in his/her assignment		

WEEK THREE: Date: _____

OBJECTIVE: To support the entry-level registered nurse in the development of skills and knowledge necessary to ensure consistently safe and competent nursing practice when caring for adults of all ages.

GOALS:

The orientee will	Date	Initials
1. Establish an effective relationship with the RN/preceptor		
2. Organize and manage the care of two patients by Day 4 of this week		
3. Perform skills according to established procedures and protocols		
4. Review secretarial functions at nursing station with unit secretary		

Figure 3.1: Sample week-to-week orientation schedule (cont.)

WEEK FOUR: Date: _____

OBJECTIVE: To support the entry level registered nurse in the development of skills and knowledge necessary to ensure consistently safe and competent nursing practice when caring for adults of all ages.

GOALS:

The orientee will	Date	Initials
1. Manage the care of three patients by Day 4 of this week		
2. Demonstrate effective organizational and priority-setting skills		
3. Perform skills according to established procedures and protocols		
4. Complete an admission and discharge with minimal assistance		

Source: Saint Francis Hospital and Medical Center, Hartford, CT. Reprinted with permission.

Competency-based orientation

Orientation of new graduates has changed over the years. There has been a shift from validating technical skills to competency-based validation. Under this model, your assignments and use of problem-solving skills will help you meet the requirements for a given competency. A competency-based orientation program will also

- be based on adult learning principles

- offer various learning opportunities

- address developmental needs

- allow for learner self-direction

- be outcome focused

Figure 3.2 provides an example of a competency validation form for the medical-surgical unit. Your preceptor may use a similar tool to assess your skills.

Figure 3.2: Sample skill validation form

Saint Francis Hospital and Medical Center
Center for Clinical Excellence and Professional Development
Medical/Surgical Skill Validation

Employee: _____

Preceptor: _____

Employee ID: _____

Unit: _____

Date orientation completed: _____

Competency	Validation			
	Simulation in lab	On the unit		
	Validator initials	Date	Validator initials	
RESPIRATORY ASSESSMENT				
1. Apply nasal cannula/regulate 02				
2. Apply ventimask/regulate 02				
3. Set up humidified 02				
4. Trach care/change inner cannula				
5. Suction tracheostomy				
6. Suction nasotracheal				
CARDIOVASCULAR ASSESSMENT				
1. Monitor for orthostatic changes				
2. Place patient on cardiac monitor				
GASTROINTESTINAL ASSESSMENT				
1. Hemetest stool				
2. Change ostomy appliance				
3. Diarrhea management				
GENITOURINARY ASSESSMENT				
1. Bladder scan for residual				
2. Assess for signs of UTI				
3. Monitor urinary output/shift				
4. Assess fluid balance status				
5. Straight catheterization-female				
6. Straight catheterization-male				
7. Indwelling catheterization-male				
8. Indwelling catheterization-female				
9. Texas condom cath				

Competency	Validation			
	Simulation in lab	On the unit		
	Validator initials	Date	Validator initials	
NEUROLOGICAL ASSESSMENT				
Neuro checks/document				
Cognition/confusion assessment				
Functional assessment				
MEDICATION ADMINISTRATION				
Administers meds per hospital policy				
IV piggyback				
IV push				
Syringe pump				
Feeding tube				
Intermittent peripheral				
Intermittent central access				
Orientation to PYXIS use				
IV FLUID MANAGEMENT				
Prepare and hang IV bag				
Regulate flow off infusion pump				
Inspect site and document				
Schedule IV site change per policy				
Baxter pump				
Colleague pump				
Document fluids on I+O sheet				
CENTRAL LINE				
Maintain patency of ports				
TLC dressing change				
Obtain blood samples				
Inspect site and document				
Remove TLC				

Source: Saint Francis Hospital and Medical Center, Hartford, CT. Reprinted with permission.

Addressing concerns

Those healthcare organizations that recognize the true functional level of a new graduate in his/her first year will have an excellent orientation program that extends beyond the traditional 3–4 months. In fact, they will strive to keep you with your preceptor for as long as you think necessary.

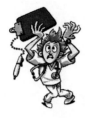

Don't panic: Along the way, you may feel anxious and stressed, but you are not alone. Many of your peers are feeling the same way. Your stress may be due to your lack of confidence in your clinical skills, or to feelings of work overload. You may have disappointment over the inability to give nursing care the way you did as a student nurse. You may feel anxious about making a mistake that could harm a patient, or you may lack knowledge and skills about patient care that cause you to be unsure of your clinical decisions.

These concerns are natural and part of the learning process. A good orientation program will address these issues and provide you with practical ways to face your fears and grow into the best nurse that you can be.

> *"I didn't expect that there would be as many decisions—you know, critical thinking at the bedside and putting it all together."*
> –2006 Graduate

What's your learning style?

In order to maximize your learning during the orientation phase and beyond, you first need to know what your learning style is and how you learn best. By understanding your learning style, you will be able to discuss this with your preceptor and nurse educator so that they can ensure a good outcome by the end of your orientation. Take a look at Figure 3.3 to see what learning style you favor. Don't worry if you find that you use a combination of learning styles—most adult learners do.

Figure 3.3: Summary of learning styles

Style	Characteristics
Visual learners (30%–40% of all learners)	• Learn by "looking" • Prefer passive surroundings • Like handouts, computer programs, etc., that are colorful and well illustrated • Enjoy the classroom setting and verbal discussions that contain a lot of imagery • Are distracted by too many auditory stimuli • Like to close their eyes and visualize what they're learning
Auditory learners (20%–30% of all learners)	• Learn by hearing • Prefer audiotapes, lectures, and discussions • Respond best to verbal instructions • Reveal emotions by changes in the tone and quality of their speech • Talk through problems and procedures and express solutions verbally
Kinesthetic learners (30%-50% of all learners)	• Learn by physical activity and direct, hands-on involvement • Learn best by "doing" • Can't sit still for long periods of time • Speak with their hands • Remember what activities are demonstrated, but have trouble remembering what was said • Enjoy skill demonstration and return demonstration

Source: Avillion, A. 2006. Designing Nursing Orientation: Evidence-Based Strategies for Effective Programs. Marblehead, MA: HCPro, Inc.

The five key elements of a good orientation program

While orientation programs vary widely from facility to facility, the best and most successful programs share similar components. Keep an eye out for the following five elements at your institution.

Element #1: Orientation information is shared

The first day of orientation should make you feel welcomed and well-treated. But before you even accept the position, you should know what your orientation will entail. During your interview, you should have received information or details about the hospital's orientation program and structure.

 Ask: If you did not receive this information, it may be beneficial for you to make a follow-up call to the facility (before you begin work) and ask:

- How long is the orientation program?

- How many days are spent in the classroom?

- How many days are spent on the unit with a preceptor?

- How do new graduates receive feedback concerning their progress?

- Is it possible to receive more time at the end of the usual orientation time if needed?

Element #2: The program is structured and comprehensive

The orientation program should be complete and organized, and have clear objectives for the training that will be taking place. It should be at least one year in length.

The level of responsibility and accountability the new graduate is expected to meet during the orientation period should closely mirror his/her function level. As a new graduate, you should feel challenged in your new position, but not completely overwhelmed by expectations.

 Don't forget: A good orientation program will strive to meet the objectives presented in your learning packet, as well as any other objectives you feel you can reasonably accomplish. **Remember, learning is a life long process.** In nursing, it is critical to remain competent in order to provide safe patient care.

Element #3: Feedback is provided throughout the program

For you to be successful, you should be evaluated frequently to ensure that your identified learning needs were met. Though the best feedback will probably come through your daily experiences, nurse educators and your preceptor should meet with you on a weekly basis to discuss your progress. Skill checklists and evaluation forms will help you see the strengths you already possess, as well as the competencies you need to develop.

At the end of your orientation, your preceptor should fill out a complete evaluation of your performance. The form may look similar to Figure 3.4.

Figure 3.4: Sample orientation summary evaluation

Saint Francis Hospital and Medical Center
Department of Patient Care Services
Center for Clinical Excellence and Professional Development

Orientation summary evaluation

Employee: _____   Employee ID:_____
Orientation end date: _____   Unit: _____

	Performance criteria	Met	Unmet
1.	Performs and accurately documents initial assessment upon arrival to the unit. Completes Admission Database within eight hours of admission.		
2.	Reviews medical history and progress notes incorporating pertinent data under "Nursing Communications" in CIS.		
3.	Initiates appropriate referrals to other disciplines based upon patient needs identified in the admission process.		
4.	Collaborates with the physician about the multidisciplinary care plan. Initiates new orders in a timely fashion.		
5.	Performs and documents a physical assessment on assigned patients at the beginning of the shift.		
6.	Establishes logical priorities and expectations based on patient's age, physical, psychosocial, and spiritual needs.		
7.	Recognizes deviations from the plan of care and/or changes in patient status.		
8.	Notifies physician of changes in a patient's condition within an appropriate timeframe.		
9.	Initiates communication with patient/family supporting the individual needs of both.		
10.	Utilizes effective communication skills that demonstrate an understanding of the communication process, resulting in information sharing, trust, and positive group dynamics.		
11.	Accepts accountability for making decisions related to patient care and works with the health team to resolve clinical problems.		
12.	Delegates activities to members of the healthcare team within their scope of practice, utilizing respectful communication, guidance, and follow up on designated responsibilities.		
13.	Provides patient/family education and referrals to supportive services.		
14.	Reprioritizes plan of care based on changing patient needs.		
15.	Demonstrates the ability to organize and manage a five-patient assignment of mixed complexity.		
16.	Completes and/or ensures that ADLs for assigned patients are met in a timely manner.		
17.	Documents on all forms in accordance with departmental standards and procedures.		

Figure 3.4: Sample orientation summary evaluation (cont.)

	Performance criteria	Met	Unmet
18.	Safely performs all clinical procedures including medication administration in accordance with established procedures/policies/protocols.		
19.	Knows the purpose, desired effect, age-specific consideration for administration and possible adverse reactions for drugs administered.		
20.	Manages the care of an unstable patient with the assistance of the preceptor.		
21.	Ensures discharge planning is completed prior to the patient leaving the hospital.		
22.	Seeks resources/consultation when needed to support and enhance knowledge and skill development.		
23.	Recognizes and accepts responsibility for achieving clinical competency and enhancing professional development.		
24.	Recognizes that people are the key to our success and the only way our shared goals can be achieved is through team effort.		
25.	Identifies opportunities for improvement.		

To be completed by the preceptor and used as an assessment of the fulfillment of orientation requirements. For any "not met" criteria, document an action plan that addresses how the criteria will be met.

Six month plan:

_____

_____

_____

_____

_____

Date of orientation summary evaluation: _____

Preceptor: _____

Orientee: _____

Clinical nurse specialist: _____

Nurse manager: _____

Source: Saint Francis Hospital and Medical Center, Hartford, CT. Reprinted with permission.

During orientation, nurse managers and supervisors should measure your success and progress toward clinical competence. During the interview process, you should have discussed the process of receiving feedback, as well as how often that feedback would be provided.

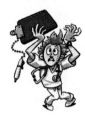

Don't panic: If you did not receive this information, you should sit down with your nurse manager and preceptor and set up a plan for obtaining feedback. It is always better to get constructive feedback in a planned manner than to wait until something happens and receive criticism that may not be as constructive as you would like. Remember: learn how to take this feedback. Listen, ask for clarification, accept the feedback graciously, and do not make excuses. You cannot improve if you don't know what you are doing wrong or how to make it right.

Element #4: Support is abundant

New graduates—like all nurses—need support from the educators, nurse managers, and staff. Their support plays a vital role in helping you make the transition from student nurse to new graduate, and also helps you deal constructively with the challenges every new nurse faces in his/her first year.

Don't forget: Support should come from a number of individuals, including

- **Nurse educators.** They understand the learning process and can help you sort out any problems you are having.

- **Nurse managers.** They understand the dynamics of the unit, including staff relations, the unit's ups and downs, and the patient population. The nurse manager is a good person from whom to seek advice on how to manage and work with other team members. But remember: If you want to receive support from your manager in regards to a staff conflict or issue, do not complain about your colleagues—instead, ask for constructive advice on how to best deal with the situation.

- **Staff.** They will be the ones who will either help or hinder your transition. It is important that you find supportive staff members because you will need them in times of stress. You may find someone on your unit or in your organization that you trust and admire—consider asking them to be your mentor.

Element #5: Orientees provide program feedback

The orientation program should continually be evaluated by the new graduates, with changes made accordingly. This feedback should include an evaluation of how the formal and unit-based orientation program met your needs, the role and effectiveness of the preceptor, and suggestions for improvement. See Figure 3.5 for a sample evaluation—your organization's form should look similar, and cover similar information. This type of form is typically completed at the end of your orientation.

The next group of orientees is sure to benefit from your honest and candid answers—you may even see the curriculum or objectives change because of your thoughtful feedback. So take the time to fill out an evaluation form, as you are making the next group of new nurses even better prepared.

Figure 3.5: Evaluation of orientation services

Evaluation of orientation services

Date: _____ Name (optional): _____

Unit/Department: _____

Preceptor: _____

Please indicate whether or not you agree with the following statements by cir-
cling the number, on a scale of 1–5, that best corresponds with your experience.
5 indicates that you strongly agree, and 1 indicates that you strongly disagree.

STAFF DEVELOPMENT SERVICES

1. Orientation classes provided by the staff development department helped me fulfill my job responsibilities.	1	2	3	4	5
2. Classroom instruction was effective and helped me meet my learning objectives.	1	2	3	4	5
3. Computer-based learning activities were effective and helped me meet my learning objectives.	1	2	3	4	5
4. Staff development specialists answered my questions satisfactorily.	1	2	3	4	5
5. Staff development specialists treated me with respect.	1	2	3	4	5

Other comments _____

_____

PRECEPTOR

1. My preceptor helped me successfully complete orientation.	1	2	3	4	5
2. My preceptor treated me with respect.	1	2	3	4	5

Figure 3.5: Evaluation of orientation services (cont.)

3. My preceptor clearly explained what was   1   2   3   4   5
    expected of me.

4. My preceptor did not ask me to perform   1   2   3   4   5
    tasks independently until I felt comfortable
    doing so.

5. My preceptor offered constructive   1   2   3   4   5
    criticism in a supportive manner and in
    a private setting.

6. My preceptor made me feel welcome.   1   2   3   4   5

Additional comments

_____

_____

_____

MANAGER AND COLLEAGUES

1. My manager clearly explained what was   1   2   3   4   5
    expected of me.

2. My manager made me feel welcome.   1   2   3   4   5

3. My manager treated me with respect.   1   2   3   4   5

4. My colleagues made me feel welcome.   1   2   3   4   5

5. My colleagues treated me with respect.   1   2   3   4   5

Additional comments

_____

_____

_____

Source: Avillion, A. 2006. Designing Nursing Orientation: Evidence-Based Strategies
for Effective Programs. _Marblehead, MA: HCPro, Inc._

Preceptor versus mentor: Why both are needed

The role of the preceptor

Precepting started in the nursing profession in the 1960s. Preceptor means "tutor." A preceptor has a formal agreement to work with a novice nurse for a specific period of time. The purpose is to ease the new graduate toward clinical competence, and assist with transition shock and staff socialization.

A preceptor's role is one of education, guidance, and supervision. He/she works with you throughout the learning process, educating you on policies and procedures and developing your competency skills. A good preceptor places your learning needs over the unit's needs. He/she also focuses on your individual growth and development during the orientation phase. For example, to foster critical thinking skills, your preceptor may test you with case scenarios, or ask you "what if" questions. If a preceptor is good at his/her role, he/she fosters an environment that encourages trust, respect, openness, values, and diversity.

Your preceptor should review your goals with you on a routine basis, as a way to ensure that your assignments are appropriate to your current function level and that you are gradually moving toward increased complexity in your work. Figure 3.6 shows what a weekly evaluation form filled out by your preceptor may look like.

Figure 3.6: Preceptor/Orientee weekly evaluation form

Date: 5/15/2006   **Week #:** 4
Preceptor: Judy Wright   **Orientee:** Kelly Kipling

Review of previous week's goals

Goal from previous week	Progress & Plan
1. Increase patient assignment # by 1 patient (min 2-3)	❑ Met ❑ Ongoing
2. Begin to incorporate all pieces for assigned patients (all meds, taking phone calls from family/MDs, documentation, etc)	❑ Met ❑ Ongoing
3. Review restraint use/skin care/pre-op or post-op procedures and documentation with preceptor	❑ Met ❑ Ongoing
4. Presents patients on plan of care rounds (Thursdays 7-3 only)	❑ Met ❑ Ongoing
5. Review PBDS with educator	❑ Met ❑ Ongoing

Plan for this week (Handwrite in from master list)

Specific objectives and experiences needed	
1. Work with chest tubes	
2. Hang blood products	
3.	
4.	
5.	

Document progress in the following areas using this scale:
1. **No experience, unaware of situation**
2. **Demonstrates awareness of situation, minimal participation, requires full guidance**
3. **Participation with moderate assistance and coaching**
4. **Performs effectively with minimal coaching**
5. **Performs effectively and independently. Aware of limitations and seeks assistance appropriately.**

Source: Hartford Hospital, Hartford, CT. Adapted and reproduced with permission.

Who makes a good preceptor?

The preceptor is the key person who will contribute to your successful completion of the orientation program. Preceptors should be those nurses who really enjoy working with new graduates, have the patience of a saint, and are well organized and able to teach.

Fact: Not every experienced nurse makes a good preceptor. There are qualities that a nurse needs to have to become a preceptor:

- Preceptors need to possess motivation and team building skills, as well as conflict resolution skills.

- Preceptors need to be able to assist the new graduate in the development of skills such as critical thinking.

- Preceptors must be able to understand the learning needs of the orientee and plan clinical experiences accordingly.

- Preceptors must be able to evaluate the orientee in a manner that encourages further learning and does not deflate the learner's self-esteem.

- Preceptors must have good communication skills, as the preceptor works with nurse educators, nurse managers, physicians, and other staff nurses.

- A preceptor should become the advocate for the new graduate in order to prevent misperceptions and isolation of the new graduate.

If a staff nurse is interested in being a preceptor, he/she should be interviewed and measured against those qualities and competencies that make a good preceptor. There should also be a formal orientation program for the preceptor. Their ongoing education should include how to be a good coach, how to work with the orientation goals set up by the education department for the new graduate, and how to help the new graduate meet the objectives and expectations of the orientation program. There should also be classes for preceptors on learning styles, adult learning principles, and effective communication strategies to help them assess and document the growth of the new graduate.

Figure 3.7: Preceptor and mentor qualities: What each can offer

Preceptor	Mentor
• Interest in teaching, mentoring and coaching • Strong communication skills • Supportive • Patient, open-minded • Able to assess if learning is taking place • Expert level of nursing • Knowledge of standards of care • Able to demonstrate the application of the nursing process when giving care	• Love and dedication to nursing • Superior communication skills • Positive outlook • Nurturing nature • Enjoyment of nursing • Demonstrated pride and respect in the profession • Strong listening skills • Trustworthy • Constructive • Collegial

The role of the mentor

Mentoring is a role that a nurse takes in order to help someone grow and learn through his/her own clinical expertise. They help with the successful transition of the new employee.

Nursing is beginning to see the need for both the preceptor and the mentor. A mentor is similar to a coach—he/she is a person you seek out and ask for support and commitment. A preceptor, on the other hand, is more like a teacher who has been assigned to you. Mentors help you in three areas:

- Workplace issues

- Professional development

- Personal growth (Zerwekh and Claborn 2006)

Who makes a good mentor?

A good mentor is someone you trust, who can guide you and who is seen as a wise person. The goal of your partnership is to help you demonstrate accountability for your actions and to grow professionally. A mentor could help you through the orientation process and into your second year of nursing practice. The mentor, however, first has to agree to be your mentor.

You can obtain a mentor in a variety of ways. At your organization, you may have a formal mentoring program, or you may consider asking a nurse in the organization who possesses the qualities that you value in a professional nurse to be your mentor. You can also talk with the nurse educator or your nurse manager and ask for help in finding a mentor based on your values and goals.

 Click: Check with professional organizations for lists of experienced nurses who are willing to mentor new nurses. Your state nurses' association may also have a list of potential mentors. In addition, there is cyber mentoring, which you can learn more about by visiting these Web sites:

- *www.nursementors-nj.com*

- *www.allnurses.com*

- *www.nursingthefuture.ca*

Extending orientation

Our greatest glory is not in never falling, but in rising every time we fall.
                                        –Confucius

If you are not progressing based on the timeframe identified by the organization, you may need an extension of your orientation to reach basic competence. Extensions are only given after thoughtful consideration of your performance and attitude. Remember, orientees are a costly investment and your orientation time was factored into the nursing budget.

Justifiable reasons for extending orientation include

- a lack of clinical progress by the new graduate

- a limited variety of patients on the unit to allow for all skills to be practiced

- the institution of new technology or courses that must be included in orientation

- the inability of the orientee to accomplish the competency goals due to lack of preceptors

If you do not demonstrate an interest or the ability to master a particular nursing specialty, consider asking for a transfer to a different unit or specialty (Mundie et al. 2005).

68

Peer support groups

Fact: In addition to a solid orientation program, the organization should offer you and your fellow new graduates a networking or support group, so that you have safe place to talk about the problems you are facing in your daily work. Studies have shown that one of the most common challenges for a new nurse is socialization into the nursing profession. But when you have an opportunity to network with your fellow new graduates, you are better able to manage work-related stressors. These support groups also help new nurses with their problem-solving skills (Herdrich and Lindsay 2006).

In the support group, you may share your feelings regarding inadequacy in your ability to practice competently, the heavy workload, conflict and conflict resolution, or any other concern you have. This safe haven gives you a chance to talk with your peers, support each other, and offer suggestions on how to successfully move through your first year.

Additional programs

The buddy system

No matter how strong your own orientation program was or how well you worked with the preceptor, you will likely encounter stress when your orientation ends. As you begin to work independently, you may encounter problems with your organizational skills, feel a lack of support, struggle with completion of your nursing tasks, and experience difficulty in upholding the quality of your work. When these issues arise, they will undoubtedly be noticed by other staff on the unit—including the shift that follows you. Some of the examples of shift-to-shift problems are

- shift report
- direct patient care issues
- follow-through on problems
- accuracy of transcription of order
- environmental checks

According to a 2005 *Journal for Nurses in Staff Development* article, one 59-bed medical-surgical unit in a community hospital started a buddy system to help alleviate this problem of the new nurse being labeled as incompetent by the unit staff. The unit identified the need for a mentoring program that included both the shift that the new graduate worked and the following shift (Guhde 2005).

Under the program, the original preceptor continues to work with the new graduate but a second nurse, on the following shift, is assigned as a "buddy" to help identify any additional problem areas with which the graduate is struggling. The buddy provides support and is expected to point out weak areas, but also to give as much positive feedback as possible (Guhde 2005).

As a result of the program, new graduates received more positive feedback and the hospital maintained a supportive learning environment. Teamwork between shifts also improved and problems needing management's attention were brought forward sooner (Guhde 2005).

If that sounds like something you'd like to be part of, consider working with your preceptor and developing a "buddy" with a nurse on the following shift. This may help you avoid the shift-to-shift strife that often plagues new graduates.

Nurse residency programs

Nurse residency programs surfaced in the 1980s. They were formed in an effort to increase the skills of the new graduate and increase recruitment and retention. Given the nursing shortage, nurse residency programs today are beneficial to both the organization and the new graduate.

It goes without saying that there is a benefit to programs that extend beyond the 3–6 month orientation program, which is what nurse residency programs do. The goal of the program is to ease the new graduate's transition into practice. Recognizing that the specific knowledge a nurse needs to become a successful, competent nurse exceeds the orientation timeframe, nurse residency programs allow the graduate nurse to expand his/her critical thinking skills in a supportive environment.

These programs usually have a standardized curriculum that integrates learning and work experiences. With a focus on quality and good outcomes, the curriculum includes evidence-based practice, patient safety standards, unit-specific clinical coursework, and communication and professional development training (Guhde 2005).

Nurse residency programs typically run for one year, and include a general orientation, preceptors, and a resident facilitator with whom to discuss issues. The resident facilitator also gives guidance in role development (Guhde 2005).

Nurse extern programs

Nurse extern programs offer student nurses the opportunity to develop their clinical skills in preparation for graduation. This program is also a recruitment tool, as it brings potential job candidates in the door and familiarizes them with the environment.

Nurse extern programs not only benefit the organization, but the student as well. The nurse extern becomes a member of the healthcare team and is not seen as just a student nurse, but as a nurse extender functioning in the role of nursing/patient care assistant. A properly structured program will encourage the extern to seek out learning experiences and make learning his/her primary focus.

Nurses at Yuma Regional Medical Center in Yuma, AZ, assign their nurse externs to a unit in which they are interested and then match each student with two preceptors: a primary and a secondary. The primary preceptor is responsible for the learning experience of the extern. The secondary preceptor serves as a resource and mentor, especially when the primary preceptor is ill or transfers to another unit. The nurse externs work along with their preceptors on three 12-hour shifts per week, including alternate weekends (Starr 2006).

Included in the 16-week summer program is a general orientation and nurse extern orientation. As in any orientation program, there is a skills checklist, weekly goals, and evaluations. Guidelines on the student's scope of practice are also reviewed (Starr 2006).

The nurse externs can provide any care for which they have demonstrated competence at their school of nursing (the only exception being medication administration and intravenous therapy). Nurse externs are expected to increase their patient workload, while always keeping their focus on learning (Starr 2006).

There are many advantages to taking part in a nurse extern program. Nurse externs

- gain basic nursing and critical thinking skills

- gain confidence

- learn to be part of a team

- build their self-confidence, thereby decreasing role stress

- are better prepared for the transition from graduate to registered nurse

References

Avillion, A. 2006. *Designing Nursing Orientation: Evidence-Based Strategies for Effective Programs.* Marblehead, MA: HCPro, Inc.

Herdrich, B., and A. Lindsay. 2006. Nurse Residency Programs: Redesigning the Transition into Practice. *Journal for Nurses in Staff Development* 22(2): 55–62.

Hom, E. 2003. Coaching and Mentoring New Graduates Entering Perinatal Nursing Practice. *Journal of Perinatal Nursing* 17(1): 35–49.

Guhde, J. 2005. When Orientation Ends: Supporting the New Nurse Who is Struggling to Succeed. *Journal for Nurses in Staff Development* 21(4): 145–149.

Lavoie-Tremblay, M. et al. 2002. How to Facilitate the Orientation of New Nurses into the Workplace. *Journal for Nurses in Staff Development* 18(2): 80–85.

McMahon, L. 2005. Mentoring: A Means of Healing New Nurses. *Holistic Nursing Practice* Sep/Oct: 195–196.

Mundie, J. et al. 2002. Orientation Outcomes in 2000 and Beyond: An Educational and Financial Partnership. *Journal for Nurses in Staff Development* 18(5): 241–247.

Starr, K., and V. Conley. 2006. Becoming a Registered Nurse: The Nurse Extern Experience. *Journal of Continuing Education in Nursing* 37(2): 86–92.

Zerwekh, J., and J. Claborn. 2006. *Nursing Today: Transition and Trends.* St. Louis: Saunders Elsevier.

Chapter 4

Transitioning from student nurse to RN

> *Knowledge comes, but wisdom lingers.*
> –Alfred Lord Tennyson

Changing roles

As you walk into your first job, you are stepping into a new role: You are now a graduate nurse (GN) or RN (if you passed your NCLEX exam). The success of this transition is up to you. The work environment will have high, and at times, unrealistic expectations of you. You need to remember that for at least the first year, you are still in transition.

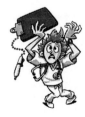 **Don't panic:** Coming off orientation should not be equated with competence. Many studies have identified the stresses and challenges faced by new graduates and cite that they need *at least* one year to feel skilled, comfortable, and confident in their role and in practice (Marcum and West 2004; Casey et al. 2004; Ellerton and Gregor 2003).

Addressing the difficulties of transition

A study published in the June 2004 issue of the *Journal of Nursing Administration* asked graduate nurses, "What difficulties, if any, are you experiencing with the transition from student role to the RN role?" Six overall themes emerged:

- Lack of confidence in skill performance, difficulty with critical thinking, and clinical knowledge

- Relationships with peers and preceptors

- Struggles with wanting to be more independent, but still having to be dependent on others

- Frustrations with the work environment

- Organization and priority-setting skills

- Communication with physicians (Casey et al. 2004)

Let's break each one down and talk about solutions.

Lack of confidence in skill performance, critical thinking, and clinical knowledge

This is a time-sensitive issue, meaning that as you progress in your position, this lack of confidence will begin to fade (and your skills will improve).

 Don't forget: You are in your first year of practice. You are still learning about nursing and patient care, and about yourself as a new nurse. As you polish your nursing skills, you will become more confident. And with more experience, you will increase your critical thinking skills and your nursing knowledge. Having self-doubt is natural, but don't spend too much time worrying about what you can't yet do—there is nothing wrong with you if you are applying yourself and working closely with your preceptor and colleagues.

New graduates become more confident in their abilities by the end of the first year, and you too will start to feel comfortable in your role. You are in the "novice" stage of nursing, on your way to advanced beginner. This transition from novice to advanced beginner will move you from *acting* like a nurse to really *being* a nurse.

Peer and preceptor relationships

We discussed this topic in both Chapters 2 and 3. It is important for you to know that many new graduates feel a lack of acceptance and respect from the experienced nurses on the unit. You may feel frustrated, thinking that your assigned preceptor is not understanding what you are going through. You may even think he/she is being insensitive to your need for help and skill development.

Tip: This issue can be resolved by being honest, but diplomatic, with your preceptor. Do this by requesting some time away from the work station to go over your concerns with what you have learned so far, what your goals are for the immediate future, and how he/she can help. Ask for honest feedback—maybe you are overlooking something in yourself that needs improvement that everyone else sees. Consider the conversation a professional growth opportunity.

> *"I had seven preceptors, and each one had a different style of doing things. It seemed as if I had a different preceptor every day. I finally went to my nurse manager and asked that I be assigned one preceptor."*
> –2006 Graduate

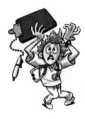

Don't panic: If, however, you feel the match between you and your preceptor is not working, you need to speak to the preceptor and explain why it is just not working for you personally. Do not focus on the shortcomings of your preceptor. Focus on your learning needs and how you are struggling to meet your goals and succeed as a new nurse. Be sure to discuss this with the nurse educator and nurse manager as well, so that they will support you and approve your request for a new preceptor.

As far as peer relationships go, your behavior, attitude, and willingness to pitch in will go a long way in winning over the staff. Find the shining star—someone who is admired by all of the team—and befriend him/her. You will learn a lot from this nurse and he/she may well be willing to be your mentor.

Next, find the nurse who is causing you problems. Ask to meet with him/her to discuss his/her perspective on how you are doing. Doing so may disarm this type of person because you are asking him/her for an opinion on how to succeed on the unit, which will be appreciated. Your goal is to convince this person to give you a chance—by showing that you value his or her help and expertise.

The struggle: Dependence versus independence

You now have a new level of responsibility. But you are not quite sure you are ready. You vacillate between wanting to prove to everyone you are indeed independent and really needing their help. It is not unusual to have this Dr. Jekyll/Mr. Hyde complex. This too is time sensitive. Chances are, you'll grow out of this complex by the end of your first year. But how do you manage this until then?

Work with everyone on the team. Build a working relationship with everyone, including the nursing assistants/patient care assistants. Good CNAs/PCAs will move mountains for a nurse who pitches in, gives them respect, and asks for their help. Don't be afraid to roll up your sleeves and get dirty, but do not fall into the trap of doing their duties in your attempt to win them over. Helping a team member when he/she really needs it is fine, but only if you are not compromising the care of your patients.

> *I cried at least a dozen times in my first year. I was overwhelmed by the patient assignment and I had to ask for help.*
> *–2005 Graduate*

Don't forget that help works both ways. When working with your colleagues, never be afraid to ask for their help before you get to the point of falling behind. At times, your colleagues will be busy with their own assignments and may not be aware that you are in need of help. Their assumption is that since you are not asking for help, you must be doing okay. When you are struggling, kindly ask others if they could help you give the pain medication in room 202, help you with a dressing change in room 216, etc. If your fellow nurses are not too busy, they will probably be glad to repay you for the favors you've done for them.

A nursing unit that promotes teamwork and sets realistic expectations for every staff member is a unit that will "pull together" when the going gets tough. Teamwork is the only way to survive in nursing today. There are too many demands and unexpected patient changes for any nurse to handle alone. As you get better at prioritizing and learning critical thinking skills, your dependence on your teammates will dwindle. And by the time the next group of new graduates arrives, you will be the one they will look to for help and support.

Frustrations with the work environment

The world of nursing is full of many stresses. This is in part due to the nature of the profession and also to the financial constraints affecting hospitals today. You may be feeling frustrated/stressed due to

- your perceptions of being overworked (often due to poor staffing)

- poor nurse-to-patient ratios

- the high expectations placed on you once orientation ends

- adjusting to your shift or working two rotating shifts

- lack of vacation time/time off from work

So how do you manage these frustrations? First, you need to understand that most of these work environment issues cannot be solved with a simple solution. You can, however, do something about them by familiarizing yourself with the environment and working for progressive change.

To start, find out what the unit budget allows for staffing based on census. Your nurse manager will know this answer. If there is a constant shortage of staff, then the problem is one that the staff and nursing management need to tackle.

 Ask: Begin by asking questions, such as these:

- Are staff members frequently calling in sick?

- Are staff members transferring to other units at the facility?

- Is turnover high?

- Is there a lack of staff members willing to pick up additional hours?

It is always best to find out the real problem and not to listen to the "grapevine." Talk to your nurse manager—you can be sure he/she is aware of the staffing issues, but may not have an immediate solution. Tell him/her your frustrations and ask if there is anything you can do to remedy the situation. By doing so, you'll show that you are interested in being part of the solution, not part of the problem.

What the team can do is brainstorm solutions to existing problems they see on the unit. A good manager will listen to the staff and have them participate in the solution. Who knows—you may have a suggestion that no one else even thought of. Now that's what we call a win-win situation!

Organization and priority-setting skills

These two skills are especially important in nursing: if you cannot prioritize the needs of the patients on your assignment, than patient care suffers; if you cannot organize your workday, than you will suffer from the stress of feeling unorganized and overwhelmed.

Not everyone is born with organizational and priority-setting skills—many of us have to learn them. "Graduates with fewer than six months of experience most often indicated that lack of organization skills seemed to be a key barrier to optimal performance in their new role" (Casey et al. 2004). These graduates find it hard to get into a routine of their own, and often feel discombobulated.

Being able to prioritize your assignment based on the patient's condition will save you time and keep your patients safe. Here is an example to help you learn how to set priorities in your daily patient care:

1. Establish a preferential order for your nursing care

    a. It must be mutual with the patient

    b. It should be based on a theoretical framework, like Maslow's hierarchy

2. Rank your priorities

    a. High-priority patients have life-threatening problems, such as loss of cardiac or respiratory function

    b. Medium-priority patients have health-threatening problems which can cause a delay in coping with physical or psychological changes

    c. Low-priority patients do not need your immediate attention (Saint Francis Hospital and Medical Center, Hartford, CT)

Figure 4.1: Priority-setting exercise

Mr. Bartlett is a 67-year-old patient on Unit 5. He had a TUR for BPH yesterday. PMHx is DVT requiring hospitalization six month ago with complete recovery. Type 1 Insulin Dependent Diabetes Mellitus. What would be your priorities for this patient at the beginning of your shift? Mark each task with the appropriate priority setting. The correct answers are provided at the end of the chapter.

H = high priority (life-threatening)
M = medium priority (health-threatening)
L = low priority

1. ___ Health teaching regarding insulin administration

2. ___ Assessing vital signs

3. ___ Ambulating the patient in the hall

4. ___ Evaluating the CBI flow both input and output

5. ___ Administering insulin

6. ___ Assessing pain level and providing pain medication

7. ___ Completing AM care

8. ___ Evaluating blood sugar level

9. ___ Completing head-to-toe rapid assessment

10. ___ Updating the Patient Care Plan including discharge plans

11. ___ Hanging the IV antibiotic due at the beginning of your shift

12. ___ Getting the shift report

Source: Saint Francis Hospital and Medical Center, Hartford, CT. Adapted and reprinted with permission.

Organization 101

Tip: A lack of organizational skills will impede your ability to get work done and finish everything properly by the end of your shift. If you find yourself struggling to put yourself and your responsibilities in order, follow these helpful hints:

- Take time to understand your assignment and PLAN YOUR SHIFT.

- Write out a timed schedule of tasks that need to be done. Make sure to prioritize those tasks so that they get done at the intended time.

- Use a worksheet to keep track of each of your patients and their needs. See Figure 4.2 for an example of a worksheet used to indicate the times and critical information for each patient at the beginning of the shift.

- Think in terms of A, B, C principles when prioritizing patient care (Airway, Breathing, Circulation).

- Think before you act. Ask yourself, "What is it that I will need when I do this procedure?"

Figure 4.2: Sample patient organizer

Room #	PT Name Age Dr.	Diagnosis & PMH	Vital Signs	Vital Signs	Diet / Activity	Labs		Report notes
Tele#			T ___ P ___ R ___ BP ___	BS ___ LS ___ O2 ___ SAT ___ BM ___				
Code status			T ___ P ___ R ___ BP ___	IV: ___			Tests	
Meds	Allergies		I ___ O ___ Foley ☐ WGT ☐	DSG △	PREC		Specimens	
Room #	PT Name Age Dr.	Diagnosis & PMH	Vital Signs	Vital Signs	Diet / Activity	Labs		Report notes
Tele#			T ___ P ___ R ___ BP ___	BS ___ LS ___ O2 ___ SAT ___ BM ___				
Code status			T ___ P ___ R ___ BP ___	IV: ___			Tests	
Meds	Allergies		I ___ O ___ Foley ☐ WGT ☐	DSG △	PREC		Specimens	
Room #	PT Name Age Dr.	Diagnosis & PMH	Vital Signs	Vital Signs	Diet / Activity	Labs		Report notes
Tele#			T ___ P ___ R ___ BP ___	BS ___ LS ___ O2 ___ SAT ___ BM ___				
Code status			T ___ P ___ R ___ BP ___	IV: ___			Tests	
Meds	Allergies		I ___ O ___ Foley ☐ WGT ☐	DSG △	PREC		Specimens	

Communication with physicians

Nurse-physician communication is an ongoing and long-standing challenge for nurses—and one that probably won't be going away anytime soon. However, there are a number of strategies you can practice to improve your communication.

Tip: The key to effective communication is being prepared before you speak. Before you call or discuss a patient problem with the physician, jot down the information that you need to relay, as well as any other important information. Know your vital signs, the lab values, and what assessment parameters made you think you needed to call. Be prepared to answer questions and try to have the answers. (If you cannot answer the physician's question, just say so, but consider it a lesson learned and be prepared the next time). Being prepared shows the physician that you are being respectful of his/her time and that you are confident and smart enough to bring the problem to his/her attention. Not only that, but you'll have much more success at getting the treatment plan you think is best for your patient.

In order to develop good working relationships with physicians, you must first gain their respect. You'll earn this through your interactions with them, as well as through the patient care that you deliver. Let's run through a scenario of how to properly and effectively communicate with a physician:

Amy's patient has had a change in condition since the previous shift report. Amy examines the patient and does the appropriate nursing interventions per protocol to minimize the patient's downward spiral. She decides to quickly discuss the patient's case with an experienced staff nurse and gives her the history and changes she assessed (e.g. vital signs, lab results, point of care test results, recent MD orders). The nurse agrees that the physician needs to be notified. Amy calls the answering service and asks Dr. Peffer to call back as soon as possible, as there has been a change in the patient's condition. When the physician calls back, Amy is prepared with her nursing assessment, nursing interventions, clinical data, and any physician orders that she used to alleviate the problem before calling.

As a result of her forethought, Amy was able to answer all of the physician's questions, and together the two were able to make a sound decision in providing the patient care.

A story of courage and confrontation

There may be times, however, when physicians step out of line and treat you with disrespect. Such behavior should not be tolerated by you, nor by anyone else on the unit. The following excerpt from *Speak Your Truth: Strategies for Effective Nurse-Physician Communication* shows how one nurse appropriately deals with such a situation.

> *Sally dreaded calling the physician. At morning rounds, he had told her that he had written prescriptions and put them in the chart. She had searched every-where and had scrutinized the chart before calling his office again. When she told him that she could not find the prescriptions, he began yelling, "I told you where they were; it's your problem, and I am not writing out more prescriptions for you." He hung up.*
>
> *Sally asked the charge nurse to help her search the patient's room and the floor and to double check that the prescriptions were not in the chart. She could not discharge the patient without the pain medication. When she called back, the physician yelled again, "I am not writing them out for you again!" This time, Sally thought, he had crossed the line.*
>
> *Sally interrupted him. "Please stop saying that. The prescriptions are not for me, they are for OUR patient, whom I am trying to help. This has nothing to do with me. I am simply trying to get our patient's medication so he can go home."*

Here is Sally's shining moment. Physician-nurse relationships will improve only to the extent that nurses change their current response. Sally broke the pattern in order for the culture of domineering physicians to become extinct. All patterns of behavior can be broken by the understanding that there is another pattern available (Bartholomew 2004).

There may also be additional areas you feel unprepared for when working with physicians. You may wonder

- What if I can't read a physician's writing?

- Who is the physician I call when no one is available?

- What do I do if I did not get the treatment plan or MD orders I think I need for my patient?

All of these are good questions. You will need to learn the answers to them during your orientation period. The unit secretary will know who is "on call," or which team is to be called. The secretary will also be able to read the physician's handwriting, as they have usually worked with the physician and worked through this same issue. Work with them as your "interpreter of MD orders." If you are having difficulty deciphering progress notes and need to document your clinical care, think SOAP, which is an acronym for **S**ubjective data (i.e., What did the patient say?), **O**bjective data (i.e., What family/work/social background information can I provide about the patient?), **A**ssessment, and **P**lan for treatment.

If you did not get the treatment plan you think you need for your patient, discuss it with the charge nurse or supervisor. They will be able to help you figure out how to care for the patient or may make a follow-up call to the physician if things are still not right.

The gap between school and the working world

Later in this book we'll talk about the reality shock that new nurses go through when they enter the "real world." For now, let's focus on the gap between what you experienced in the clinical setting and what you will be facing in the work world.

Think of this scenario: *You are on your last day of your clinical rotation and you are handling your clinical assignment like a pro. You have three patients, your preparation was easy, and now you just have to read the latest orders and progress notes. You know the medications and nursing procedures for your patients and you have already discussed each patient's plan of care with the assigned RN. You feel good about your day, which has turned out well. You are ready for graduation and feel that nursing school has prepared you well for the rigors of being a real nurse.*

Fast forward five months: *You are now an RN, working the night shift on a medical-surgical unit in a small community hospital. It is about 4:00 a.m. and your shift started at 7:00 p.m. You are working with two RNs and two PCAs on a 24-bed unit. On this particular shift, your assignment includes an 80-year-old man with CHF admitted the day before, a 54-year-old woman who had abdominal surgery that morning, a 30-year-old man in traction from an MVA, a 75-year-old female on IV antibiotics with pneumonia, and a 37-year-old man admitted for DKA and ETOH abuse. Then, the emergency department calls with a new admission for a 22-year-old with status asthmaticus.*

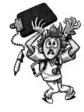

Don't panic: You now need to think on your feet and prioritize your nursing care. What would you do? The other experienced nurses are too busy for you to run your decisions by them. Wishing for more help is not an option. Neither is questioning, "Why did I go into nursing anyway?"

> *"Clinical shelters you from the realities of dealing with physicians, pharmacists, the reality of working in a hospital, and all aspects of it. When in school, everything is in a nice neat box."*
> –2005 Graduate

When the reality of nursing sinks in, you need to stay calm and develop a plan of action. Moments like this are sure to come, so you might as well prepare for them. How? By thinking about the skills you learned in school and during your orientation, and prioritizing your responsibilities. Look at your patients now and delegate appropriately so that you can manage the new admission. If you are organized and keep up with your tasks and documentation, you will be able to work safely and efficiently.

After the shift, debrief with the other nurses or someone you have chosen as a mentor. Talk about what went right and what went wrong. What did you learn from this experience? Remember, every experience can be a "lesson learned."

New grad worries: You are not alone

If there is one theme in this book, it is that all new graduates have common worries, challenges, and stress—no matter which country or school of nursing they graduated from.

Most new graduates ask themselves

- Did I pick the right unit?

- How do I get the most out of orientation?

- Will I learn enough?

- How will I work with families?

- How will I work with physicians?

- What about the different shifts?

- Will I have free time outside of work?

- How will I manage work, home, family, and friends?
  (Steinmiller et al. 2003)

Tip: All of the above concerns are valid, but the idea is to not let a concern become a stressor or breaking point for you. This is where some of the strategies mentioned earlier come into play. Find a mentor and discuss some of the issues you're having—most nurses asked themselves the same questions when they started. Find a peer or start a new grad support group. It does not have to be a formal one. Maybe it's just coffee or drinks after work once a week. Peer-to-peer time of any kind is priceless, especially during the transitional first year. Listen to your teammates, and ask them how are they managing their hectic schedules and coping with their experiences—their stories may provide you with some of the answers you've been looking for.

The unavoidable meltdown

You have completed your orientation and are now practicing alone. Your preceptor is still available, but no longer "assigned" to you. Your workload is getting more difficult. You feel yourself getting more and more anxious about going to work. Then, during your shift, you have a "meltdown." You are not alone. As you'll see from the following nurse manager's experience, this phenomenon is not only natural, but common:

"I have been a nurse manager for about 12 years at a teaching institution. Over the years I have hired a large number of new nurses. There is this magical period when they have a 'meltdown'—almost every nurse I have hired has had this melt-down around the third or fourth month after starting to work as a nurse. I have seen it in both types of new nurses: the ones who lack confidence in themselves and don't think they will ever be smart enough to do all that the preceptor can do, and

the ones who know everything. We tell them that all new nurses have a 'meltdown' and to expect it. It is a normal process of growing up in nursing. Just take a step back, catch your breath, and go back to what your learning needs are."

Clinical competency

Competence in nursing has been defined as the nurse's ability to demonstrate a predetermined set of skills within a set timeframe. Nurses develop in stages of competence. Based on Patricia Benner's work, a nurse is considered competent after being in practice for 18 months to two years (Benner 1984). Her framework for identifying the stages of nurse competence is illustrated in the following chart.

Figure 4.3: Benner's levels of nursing skill development

Stage	Description
Novice	• Does not have previous experience in the clinical situation • Task-oriented • Needs rules to perform safely
Advanced Beginner	• Experience with enough situations that he/she can demonstrate limited, but acceptable, clinical skill • Begins to make a connection between foundational knowledge of the clinical situation and identification of the patient's needs • Needs assistance from preceptors
Competent	• Has been on the job in the same or similar situation for 2-3 years • Consistently applies critical thinking skills to identification of actual and potential problems • Can formulate an appropriate plan of care • Has a wide knowledge base and an increased level of efficiency
Proficient	• Able to see the entire clinical picture for the patient • Can draw from previous experience and knowledge to determine whether the patient falls within the expected clinical course
Expert	• Has extensive background and experience • Uses intuitive capability to identify a problem • Does not waste time with unfruitful, alternative diagnoses and solutions

Source: Benner, P. 1984. From Novice to Expert: Excellence and Power in Clinical Nursing Practice. Menlo Park, CA: Addison-Wesley.

We can use Benner's model in the new-graduate learning process. As a new graduate, you need to learn how to develop therapeutic relationships with patients and families, organize their patient care, and develop relationships with other healthcare team members. In your novice experience, many of these lessons will be learned through "event markers," or situations that leave a professional impact on your career. Such experiences are unavoidable and not always pleasant (e.g., dealing with a disruptive patient), but they will undoubtedly prepare you for what's to come.

The novice stage: How to manage it

Have patience with all things, but chiefly have patience with yourself.
Do not lose courage in considering your own imperfections,
but instantly set about remedying them—everyday a task anew.
–St. Francis DeSales

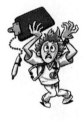

Don't panic: The novice stage of nursing is one filled with tremendous on-the-job learning, as you begin integrating what you learned in school with what the job demands. Give yourself time to grow into the "advanced-beginner" stage; this should happen naturally as you deal with more patients/ families, improve your organizational, communication, and collaboration skills, and endure your first significant event markers.

Figure 4.4: New-graduate transition and stages of competence

	Novice: First 3 months	Beginner: 4–12 months	Advanced beginner: 13–18 months
Patient and family	• Learning new procedures • Perfecting skills • Follows standards of care • Sees patient conditions as challenges	• Fear of patients asking questions they cannot answer	• Family seen as a new demand • Comfortable with procedures
Organization skills	• Struggles with being organized during shift	• Shift organization improving	• Organization has improved • Others have noticed improvement
Working with the team	• Dependent on the team • Needs preceptor • Fear of team talking about them • Approach MDs with reluctance	• Beginning to integrate into team • Physician communication still a problem	• Unit is "home" • Still concerned with staffing levels • MD relationship still a problem, but sees value in building collaborative relationship
Marker events	• First patient death • First error • Development of new skills	• Know the answer to questions asked by other staff	• May be asked to be a preceptor • Compares self to new graduates • Able to get out on time • May assume charge nurse responsibilities

During the novice stage, it's crucial that you know the rules of the unit and of the type of patient care that is expected. You should have reviewed policies, protocols, and standards of care during your orientation—don't forget them, as understanding the system is an essential element of competence. Why must you follow the formal rules and policies of the unit? Because they are not only the rules that govern safe and effective nursing care, they will also help you maneuver through your first months post-orientation.

Standards of care

Standards of care represent a level of nursing care that is expected of any nurse caring for any particular patient. Consider it a recipe for success. Just like making a cake, there are basic ingredients needed, like vital signs, physical assessments based on the patient's presentation, ambulation after surgery within a set timeframe, patient education, etc. You can add your own creative ingredients as well, like the way in which you conduct your patient/family education, or your own therapeutic nurse-patient relationship techniques, but the basic ingredients always remain the same.

 Watch out: If the recipe is not followed and we vary from this basic standard of care, there will be a variance in the patient's outcome. Maybe we will see a post-op pneumonia because we did not use the incentive spirometer, or auscultate breath sounds, or ask the patient to turn, cough, and take deep breaths. Remember that set interventions exist for a reason, and they will help you remember what is expected and needs to be done at a minimal level.

Once you become comfortable with the standard of care for each diagnosis on your unit, you will not only be able to employ the basic requirements of care, but go beyond those requirements and incorporate other appropriate nursing interventions—kind of like adding fruit and nuts to your cake recipe.

Protocols

Your organization's protocols are another area that should have been covered during orientation. They are necessary for any given nursing intervention. An organization committed to patient safety and quality outcomes will have written protocols for every nurse to follow. If you learn and follow them, you will never be in a position of legal liability.

You will not be expected to memorize every protocol. However, to ensure that you are delivering safe patient care, you will be expected to know where to find particular protocols with which you may not be familiar. The following is an example of how a new nurse correctly followed protocol.

*Mary was working with a patient with chest tubes. She remembered her compe-
tency skills from nursing school, but wanted reassurance that she was going to
do the right thing. She discussed turning the regulator on the wall down to
decrease the suction and pressure with Joan, a 15-year nurse veteran.*

"That's not how you do it. You have to use the pleurovac valve," Joan said.

*Remembering information she learned in school, Mary questioned Joan's sugges-
tion. "You know, Joan, you may be right, but I would feel more comfortable if I
looked it up in the protocol manual because I am still new at this. I hope you
don't mind."*

*Mary consulted the hospital's protocol manual—her initial decision to turn
down the suction regulator was correct.*

*During her new nurse group meeting that week, Mary mentioned what hap-
pened with the nurse educator. The nurse educator commended her on following
protocol and not being pressured to compromise patient care.*

 Don't forget: As you can see, you will be openly challenged as a new
graduate. In this case the "rules" of nursing practice (i.e., protocol) worked
in Mary's favor. She also used her novice status to her advantage by identifying that she wanted to do the right thing. And doing the right thing can
never be wrong in the eyes of others.

The above example demonstrates some of the challenges you will face working with different team members. Keep in mind we are all different in our
personalities, culture, and communication styles. You will need to learn
effective communication skills to successfully integrate into your workplace.
Yes, there will be times when someone will make you feel incompetent. At
those moments, you need to step back and assess the situation. Reflect on
what happened and formulate a plan on how to address the issue and
those involved.

Working with the team

How do you develop your communication skills? First, when you are communicating an issue, be thoughtful in your approach, tone, and in the words
you use. The old adage, "Think before you speak" is a good one to remember.

The basic principles of effective communication

Communication is not just words—it is an art that must be mastered in order for you to be understood and to understand others.

Tip: Keep the following principles in mind:

1. Communication is a process involving interaction between at least two persons. Giving a report is not communication unless you give the person receiving the report time to respond.

2. You hold the responsibility of making your message as clear as possible. It is okay to say, "I want to be sure I gave you the right information. Can you tell me what I said?"

3. Simple, concise words provide clarity and prevent misunderstanding.

4. Your body language also conveys a message.

5. People listen more carefully to those they respect—strive to develop a reputation of being trustworthy, reliable, and competent.

6. Build positive relationships with everyone on your team. Acknowledge others' feelings, needs, and contributions.

7. Always communicate with the person you want to receive your message. Remind yourself to "send the mail to the right address" and not down other avenues. To become trusted, talk to the person you need to when a problem arises—not anyone else.

8. Keep your personal values and biases in check (Zerwekh and Claborn 2006).

There will be times as a professional nurse when someone will attack you verbally. Regardless of whether it was warranted or not, you are entitled to the same respect that you show others. You need to learn how to address and resolve conflict in a positive way. We will discuss this issue in more depth in Chapter 8.

There are many resources, such as nursing journals and reference books, that deal with communication and conflict resolution. A great way to be prepared is to have a peer role play the interaction with you. Practicing conflict-resolution techniques will help you become more comfortable in managing conflict. And remember: developing a professional communication style is a learning process—it doesn't happen overnight.

Managing conflict: Helpful hints

Tip: If you find yourself in a contentious situation, try defusing the situation with some of the following techniques:

- Maintain an open and empathetic tone of voice.

- Maintain eye contact (unless this would be perceived as culturally insensitive).

- Maintain an open body stance. Do not cross your arms.

- Do not back away unless you think you will be in danger.

- Try and have the discussion moved to a private location.

- Listen and do not interrupt.

- Avoid becoming defensive.

- Focus on the problem and not the person.

- Use "I" messages such as "I thought that . . ." or "I believe . . ."

- Stay away from judgmental or inflammatory words.

- Repeat what you believe you are hearing, such as "I think you are saying ____. Is that correct?" (Cherry and Jacob 2005)

Achieving competence and confidence

> *Nursing is a combination of head, heart, and hands. Once you develop all three you will be a competent nurse.*
>
> –P. Duclos-Miller

In order to show that you are a competent nurse, you will have to question your environment, question clinical judgment, and begin to make sense out of a chaotic environment. As a new graduate, however, you will be very task-oriented and focused on developing your technical skills. The goal is for you to transition from a task-oriented mindset to a patient-outcome-focused level of care (Marcum and West 2004).

Watch out: Worried that you'll never become a competent nurse? Sometimes you can be your own worst enemy. You have so much self-doubt that you develop a defeatist attitude. To stop this self-destruction you need to stop

- overgeneralizing

- jumping to conclusions

- mind reading

- personalizing every problem (e.g., "It's my fault," "They're talking about me.")

- all-or-nothing thinking (e.g., "If don't do this perfectly, I'll never be a good nurse")

Begin focusing on the positive. Use "self affirmations" in the form of sticky notes: find a phrase or "pearls of wisdom" that inspire you and stick them on your work locker, in your car, and around your home. Think of Yoda in the *Star Wars* series who told Luke Skywalker, "Try not. Do or do not. There is no try." Before going to work, think about the positive ways you will handle a crisis. By being proactive rather than reactive, and by making frequent rounds on your patients, you may even stop a crisis before it occurs. Not only that, but you'll begin showing others just how competent you are.

Competency is a combination of many professional characteristics, including emotional intelligence, intellectual capability, profession-specific skills and knowledge, and generic skills and knowledge. Here is a self assessment to test where your level of competence is today. Remember to come back every few months and take it again.

Figure 4.5: Professional capability scale

Key: C = Competent			NI = Need improvement NAY = Not acquired yet
C	**NI**	**NAY**	**Emotional intelligence-personal**
			I am willing to face and learn from my errors, and listen openly to feedback.
			I understand my personal strengths and limitations.
			I am confident enough to take calculated risks.
			I can remain calm when things go wrong.
			I can wait, think it out, and not jump in too quickly to resolve a problem.
			I want to produce as good a job as possible.
			I am willing to pitch in and undertake menial tasks when needed.
			I have a sense of humor and can keep work in perspective.
			Emotional intelligence-interpersonal
			I can empathize with and work productively with people from a wide range of backgrounds.
			I am willing to listen to different points of view before coming to a decision.
			I am able to develop and use my colleagues to help me solve key workplace problems.
			I can work with senior staff without being intimidated.
			I can give constructive feedback to colleagues without using blame.
			I am able to develop and contribute positively to team-based projects.
			Intellectual capability
			I know that there is never a fixed set of steps for solving workplace problems.
			I can use previous experience to problem solve when a current situation takes an unexpected turn.
			I am able to diagnose what is really causing the problem and use the correct nursing action(s).
			I can readjust a plan of action depending on how the patient/situation turns out.
			I can set and justify priorities.
			Profession-specific skills and knowledge
			I have a high level of current technical expertise in nursing. (This would be expected of an "expert" level nurse.)
			Generic skills and knowledge
			I can use information technology to communicate and perform key work functions.
			I am able to organize my work and manage time effectively.
			I can manage my own ongoing professional learning and development.
			I have the ability to help others learn in the workplace.
			I understand how an organization such as mine operates.

Source: Adapted from Rochester, S. et al. 2005. Learning from success: Improving undergraduate education through understanding the capabilities of successful nurse graduates. Nurse Education Today *25: 181-188.*

See yourself as evolving or "a work in progress." Becoming a competent nurse takes time and experience. Have confidence in yourself. Give yourself time. And never lose sight of the reason you wanted to become a nurse. You are a valued member of the profession.

The following is a story to help you along the way.

A well-known speaker started off his seminar by holding up a $20 dollar bill. He asked the audience, "Who would like this $20 bill?" Hands started going up.

"I am going to give this $20 to one of you, but first, let me do this," he said. He proceeded to crumple the bill. He then asked, "Who still wants it?" Hands still went up.

"Well, what if I do this?" he asked, dropping the bill on the floor and then grinding it with his shoe. He picked it up, now crumpled and dirty. "Now, who still wants it?" Hands still went up.

He told the audience that they had all learned a very valuable lesson. "No matter what I did to the money, you still wanted it because it did not decrease in value. It was still worth $20."

Many times in nursing you will feel dropped, crumpled, and stepped on. You will feel as though you are worthless. But not matter what has happened or what will happen, you will never lose your value. Dirty or clean, crumpled or finely creased, you are still priceless to all of us in nursing. You are the nurses of the future. Be proud of that!

Priority-setting exercise answers:

1. L
2. M
3. M
4. M
5. H
6. M
7. L
8. H
9. H
10. L
11. M
12. L

References

Bartholomew, K. 2004. *Speak Your Truth: Proven Strategies for Effective Nurse-Physician Communication.* Marblehead, MA: HCPro, Inc.

Benner, P. 1984. *From Novice to Expert: Excellence and Power in Clinical Nursing Practice.* Menlo Park, CA: Addison-Wesley.

Casey, K. et al. June 2004. The Graduate Nurse Experience. *Journal of Nursing Administration* 34(6): 303–311.

Cherry, B., and S. Jacob. 2005. *Contemporary Nursing Issues, Trends and Management.* St. Louis: Elsevier Mosby.

Ellerton, M. and R. Gregor. 2003. A Study of Transition: The New Nurse Graduate at 3 Months. *The Journal of Continuing Education in Nursing* 34(3): 103–107.

Marcum, E., and R. West. 2004. Structured Orientation for New Graduates: A Retention Strategy. *Journal for Nurses in Staff Development* 20(3): 118–124.

Rochester, S. et al. 2005. Learning from success: Improving undergraduate education through understanding the capabilities of successful nurse graduates. *Nurse Education Today* 25: 181–188.

Saint Francis Hospital and Medical Center. Hartford, CT.

Steinmiller, E. et al. 2003. Rx for Success: A conference addresses 'reality shock' with future nurses. *American Journal of Nursing* 103(11): 64A–64B.

Zerwekh, J., and J. Claborn. 2006. *Nursing Today: Transition and Trends.* St. Louis: Saunders Elsevier.

Chapter 5

Overcoming reality shock

A whole new world

Just as people from foreign countries experience culture shock when they arrive in the United States, new nurses struggle with reality shock when they first enter the world of nursing. For foreigners, American culture can be very different from their own, especially in terms of societal norms, language, and interaction. It takes time to become familiar with one's new surroundings and "fit in."

As a new graduate, you probably have experienced many of these same feelings. In your new job, you have to get used to the norms of the unit and how members of the team interact with one another. You need to learn additional medical and nursing language to communicate effectively. You must familiarize yourself with your unit's physical plant, medication, and charting systems, all of which are new to you. And on top of all that, you need to adapt to your new role and fit into the team.

"I was scared to go into my patient's room—it was like the first day of clinical."
                                                                    –2005 Graduate

You are on your own and starting a new role. Your fellow student nurses and your clinical instructor are gone. You will now be assessed and judged by the patient care assistants, physicians, the unit secretary, and everyone else on your new team. There will be times when you question yourself because the real world of nursing is nothing like the clinical lab world of nursing school. There will be a big difference between what you will see and do on the unit and what you learned in school. Nursing school may have helped you with your practical skills, but you will find that nursing school really gives you nursing theory—what you find in the real world may be completely different.

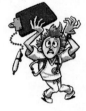

Don't panic: The goal of this chapter is to help you identify what "reality shock" is and how to manage it so that you can become a successful new nurse. Reality shock does not last forever. In time, you will learn how to integrate your "ideal world" into your "real world."

Reality shock: What is it?

Reality shock can be defined as *"a condition that exists when a person prepares for a profession, enters the profession, and then finds that he or she is not prepared"* (Cherry and Jacob 2005).

Reality shock is not unique to nursing. All professionals face it when they leave the academic world and enter the working world. You probably discussed the transition stages of reality shock during your last year of nursing school. The faculty member who presented this material was trying to prepare you for the "culture shock" that all new graduates face—it is simply part of the experience of moving from an expert student nurse to a novice professional nurse. The following is my own experience as a new graduate.

I started my nursing career the day after I graduated. I soon realized that I needed to "think" on my own. There was no instructor off whom I could bounce my ideas about patient care, and there were no fellow students to help me with nursing tasks. In those days, we were doing team nursing, so the RN was in charge of the LPNs and CNAs. I was given a full assignment within two weeks. The unit had an efficient nursing staff and a working head nurse. It seemed as if they were able to manage their assignment effortlessly. I felt as if I was working in slow motion.

I was the first BSN hired onto the unit and felt as if the weight of all BSN graduates was on my shoulders. I needed to prove that we were as good as the diploma nurses. There was a former army nurse who made it clear she did not like BSN graduates. She said that we did not get enough clinical time to become good nurses and that she was not about to finish my education on how to become one. She had her meds, assignments, AM care, and beds finished by coffee break. Yes, she seemed like a robot doing "tasks," but I watched her and I learned a lot from her. During my first year I learned vital nursing skills, task/time management, and the art of caring.

The phases of reality shock

Nurse researcher Marlene Kramer, RN, PhD, FAAN, studied the transition from student nurse to new-graduate nurse and found that there are four phases of reality shock: the honeymoon phase, the shock (rejection) phase, the recovery phase, and the resolution phase (Kramer 1974).

Figure 5.1: Kramer's four phases of reality shock

Honeymoon	Shock (Rejection)	Recovery	Resolution
• Nursing is the best. • I am finally a nurse. • I am on my own. • I want to be respected.	• Who do I believe? • I am so tired. • What is wrong with me? I am so stupid. • What is wrong with them? • They don't care about the right way to do it.	• Something funny happened today. • I think they like working with me. • I can do that. • I know what is "good" and "bad" care.	• My nurse manager says I am doing well. • I know how to balance what I learned with what to do at work.

Source: Kramer, M. 1974. Reality Shock: Why nurses leave nursing. *St. Louis: Mosby.*

The honeymoon phase

During this phase, you are delighted to be a new nurse. It is everything that you imagined. You are still in orientation and meeting other new graduates. Everyone in the group is excited about their choice to become a nurse. But this phase is short-lived.

> *"After two weeks, my honeymoon phase was over."*
> —2006 Graduate

Soon, you begin to see the differences between what you learned in school and what is really going on. You wonder which set of values you are supposed to uphold—the ones you learned in school, or the ones that every other nurse on your unit is using. These feelings eventually lead you into the second phase—shock. You may become angry that you must compromise what you've been taught in order to survive. Your self-esteem may begin to falter as you become hypercritical of yourself and of nursing.

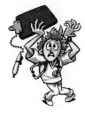

Don't panic: If you feel like you're in this phase, don't fall into the trap—nursing needs you. The key to moving out of this phase is the right attitude. Convince yourself that you have what it takes, and bear in mind that things will get easier. Dig deep inside and remind yourself why you wanted to become a nurse.

The shock (rejection) phase

Your orientation program is over and you are now working on your own. You get your own assignment and have to complete your own nursing tasks. When you ask a more-seasoned staff nurse about a particular task, you get an answer that does not match what you learned in school. Or, you may get a "Because that's the way we do it here" response.

> *"Be careful—there will be a temptation to use short cuts,*
> *but know what the repercussions can be. I've seen nurses*
> *give tube feedings without checking for placement."*
> —2006 Graduate

Your head spins as you look for your clinical support, preceptor, or instructor and realize that you are not a student nurse anymore and must stand on your own two feet. You are doing the best that you can but still feel as though you do not accomplish anything. You begin to wonder how your fellow students are doing and wish you could be back in school.

During this phase, you may feel a bit like each of the following types of nurses, which is natural during your first months on the job. Consider yourself a work in progress.

- **The native.** These nurses decides they cannot fight the seasoned nurses and join in the way they do things. They begin to take shortcuts, even when they compromise patient safety (e.g., not looking up medications with which they are unfamiliar).

- **The runaway.** They decide to "run away" from the profession because it is too difficult/not what they expected.

- **The appliance.** These nurses decide to do just what is needed to get by. We call these nurses "appliance nurses" because they only work to get new appliances and other material things.

- **The burn-out.** These nurses keep their feelings and internal conflict to themselves. They burn out because they do not manage stress effectively, and/or take on too many responsibilities. They begin to feel tired all the time, have frequent headaches, difficulty sleeping, mood swings, and anxiety. Ultimately, the quality of their work (and health) suffers.

- **The loner.** They decide to just keep quiet and do the job.

- **The new nurse on the block.** These nurses decide to change jobs whenever the work environment does not meet their needs. They are always the newest member of the team.

- **The change agent.** These nurses decides that it is better to stay and work with the system to make the changes necessary. They go to their nurse managers with suggestions on how to improve things (Kramer 1974).

Ask: During the shock phase, Kramer suggests you ask yourself two important questions:

1. What must I do to become the nurse I really want to be?
2. What must I do so that my nursing contributes to my patients and the community?

By answering these questions, you will get a better grip on your priorities and on the path you must follow to become the best nurse you can be.

So what type of nurse do you really want to become? Look around you, find those nurses whose qualities you admire, and try to emulate them. They will appreciate your effort to improve.

> *"Remember to be open-minded to changes and a different way of doing something—as long as it is a safe way."*
> –2006 Graduate

The recovery phase

Humor is the first sign of this phase. You begin to see things in a positive light and stop taking everything so seriously. There is now a balance between the ideal and the real world. You begin to understand the culture of nursing. You can differentiate between the good and the bad of the work world. You are less stressed and anxious, and your healing process begins. Finally, you are able to see things in your work world objectively and can communicate effectively with staff.

Tip: Suggestions to help you in this phase are to use prioritization, time management, and a support person or group. Also, focus on developing your positive conflict-resolution skills, as they will help you grow profession-ally and manage the work world. We will focus on ways to improve these skills in later chapters. Soon enough, you will begin to see that you have the capacity to change a situation.

The resolution phase

This phase comes after you have resolved the conflict between the academic and work world. You feel ready to provide quality nursing care to your patients. You finally see yourself as "part of the team." No longer do you struggle through each day—in fact, you enjoy your job and take pride in the care you give your patients.

Help is a click away

Most of you will move through each of these phases at your own pace. You will each experience reality shock differently and deal with it based on your own terms. But the important thing to remember is that you will all get through it!

Click: If you are looking for some support as you transition through the phases of reality shock, check out *www.allnurses.com/forums/realityshock*. There, you'll find an online forum for new nurses to discuss their issues during the first year of nursing. Experienced nurses give their support and suggestions as well.

What you didn't learn in school

The North Carolina Center for Nursing did a recent study of 329 new graduate nurses from across the state in an effort to evaluate their first-year experiences on the job. The new graduates identified three areas that they would have liked more focus put on during nursing school:

1. Hands-on learning
2. The real world of nursing
3. The tricks of the trade (Scott 2006)

Although you are already out of nursing school, let's address each of these areas so that you are more comfortable transitioning through the phases of reality shock and into the role of professional nurse.

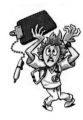

Hands-on learning
Don't panic: You may not be able to go back to the classroom, but you can use your orientation period to gain more hands-on experience. During this time, you—and everyone else on the staff—should acknowledge that you are unseasoned and need time to practice your skills.

It's okay to say that you do not know how to catheterize a male patient, or how to insert an NG tube. This is your time to learn those skills that were not taught in nursing school. It is also the time for you to practice those tasks/procedures that you do not feel comfortable doing.

Use your first few months on the job to improve your skills and your self-confidence. Let the nurse educator know what your learning needs are and what you expect to accomplish at the end of the orientation time. Keep your preceptor informed of your changing skills and learning needs, remembering to add your own learning needs to the checklist. And don't become frightened by the length of your list—tackle one thing at a time. You are not in a race.

The real world of nursing

How honest were your instructors? Did they talk about the staffing shortage, your true patient workload, the long hours, the lack of sleep, the difficulties of working with others? If they did, bravo. For those of you who did not get the whole truth, here it is: You will be getting a heavy workload, one that will vary depending on the staffing on your shift. There will be staff call-ins and large numbers of unexpected admissions with no additional help. There will be many shifts where you will not be happy with the workload. But you, like all of the nurses that came before you, will learn to take the good with the bad and grow from your tribulations.

 Don't forget: Even the most experienced nurses have "bad days." During these trying times, consult your support system. Talk to your preceptor and ask him/her how to best handle your patient assignment without feeling overwhelmed. Discuss your concerns with your mentor or a fellow nurse. Arrange for some one-on-one time with your nurse manager to get out your emotions. These individuals are your resources—use them.

If your facility offers classes or sessions on time management, transitioning issues, or other topics to help you manage your patient safely, like pharmacology, take them. Nursing is a profession of lifelong learning and you are just beginning. Now is the time to gear up and enjoy the ride (including all of its twists and turns)!

The tricks of the trade

In the North Carolina Center for Nursing study, graduates opined that nursing schools need to share the "tricks" staff nurses use to survive in the hectic work environment. Here is a list of the tricks graduates said they needed:

- Priority setting

- Delegation

- Time management

- Stress management

- Positive coping strategies

- Organizational skills

- Conflict resolution skills (Scott 2006)

Let's briefly go over each of these and discuss how you can make each trick work in your favor.

Priority setting

This will help you stay out of trouble and manage your workload. When you learn how to choose which patients need to be seen first, you avoid the potential for patient complications. Follow the **A** (airway), **B** (breathing), **C** (circulation) principles of patient care and you will be fine—i.e., any patient with airway problems is first on your list, followed by any patient with breathing problems, and then any patients with circulation problems.

Delegation

You cannot do everything for all of your patients yourself. Working with the ancillary staff and knowing what an appropriate assignment is for them will help you with your workload. Just remember the **five rights of delegation** before you delegate a task.

Ask: Ask yourself:

1. **Is this the right task to delegate?** The task should be one that is frequently repeated in the daily care of patients. It should not require your nursing assessment or judgment. It should not require complex application of the nursing process. The results should be predictable, the risk minimal, and it should be within the standard or set procedure practiced by all. If you are unsure of what you can delegate, ask for a skills checklist for the patient care assistant.

2. **Are the circumstances right?** Look at the setting and the resources available. Is it reasonable in this situation to delegate the task?

3. **Is this the right person for the job?** Are you certain that this person has the skill set or competency required to do the task safely and effectively?

4. **Did you use the right communication?** This goes back to your communication skills. Did the delegated person clearly understand you (and vice versa)? Make sure to tell them your expectations, such as the acceptable range of the patient's blood pressure and what to do if the patient varies from your set range. Use the 4 Cs approach in your communication: Be clear in what you are saying; be concise and avoid unnecessary information; be sure you are asking for something that is within the correct policy/procedure and within the state law; and be sure you were complete in your instructions.

5. Did you provide the right supervision? Even when you delegate a task, you are still responsible for monitoring, evaluating, and using nursing interventions for your assigned patients. Ancillary staff who report to you are only held to their scope of practice. You are responsible for all patient outcomes.

Time management

> *Gain control of your time, and you will gain control of your life.*
> **–Anonymous**

You will need time management in your personal and work life. One of my favorite time management tricks is to "never touch a piece of paper twice." For example, when you get your mail, open it, sort it, and throw away what you don't need. Another tip is to throw out objects that you have not used in more than six months—that way, you get rid of the clutter and don't feel like your plate is overflowing.

Effective time management will help you achieve your professional goals and meet your own needs. Managing your time is a necessity in nursing, as there will be many demands on your time. Time management will also help you with organizational skills, make you feel like you have more control, and reduce wasted time. The following are a dozen time-management tricks you can incorporate into your work style:

Tip: **Twelve tips for time management**

1. Use the 80/20 rule. Twenty percent of your effort produces 80% of the results. In other words, 80% of your nursing care will be with 20% (the sickest) of your patients.

2. Find a clinical worksheet that you like and use it to manage your patient assignments. See Figure 4.2 in Chapter 4 for a sample patient-tracking chart that you can use.

3. Keep the change-of-shift report on track. Don't waste too much time talking about incidental information instead of important facts about the patients.

4. Get organized before the shift starts. Come in early and look through the charts, new MD orders, the past two shifts' progress notes, and recent lab results.

5. Plan your shift according to patient needs. Who are your priority patients? Figure out who you need to see first, second, third, etc.

6. When entering a patient room, start off right—wash your hands and introduce yourself. Also, while you are examining the patient for over-all clinical status, look at the patient area. Do you need to get more supplies for the dressing change later?

7. After your walking rounds, decide if your first impression of priority patients is the same as when you took report. Re-organize accordingly.

8. Consider each and every time you walk into a room a "teachable moment." Use your time with the patient to reinforce safety, discharge planning, and any identified learning needs. There will be no time for structured teaching. Remember that nurses who teach every time they walk into the room get the most done.

9. Delegate non-nursing activities. This will free you up to do more with your assessments and nursing-specific tasks.

10. Never wait until the end of the shift to chart. Make your entries as you go along.

11. Consult the reference texts on your unit. If there are none, bring your own or buy a PDA and download reference material so that you do not have to hunt information down during the shift, as this is a big time waster.

12. When you are dealing with patients and families and are pressed for time, be honest and tell them, "I would really like to continue this conversation, but can I get back to you in a little while? I have some-thing urgent I need to do right now." In this way you are being polite, saying that you will get back to them and letting them know that there is something more pressing that needs your attention at the moment. But make sure you do go back later, no matter how much later. You do not want to break a trusting relationship with your patient and family.

Stress management

Don't forget: Simple strategies can be used to help you cope with the stress of being a new nurse. First, you need to take an inventory of how much time you devote to yourself each day. If it is not enough time to help you decompress, then you need to make a commitment to yourself that you are worth spending time on. Use this time to get yourself back on track and focused on the future, not what has happened in the past. Remember that caring for yourself is first and foremost, as no one else will do it for you.

Next, do the things you really like. Read a chapter every day of a book that is not a text book. Take a nice relaxing bath or shower. Go for a bike ride or walk. Find a hobby that will take your mind off work. During work, if you begin to feel stressed, find a quiet room and just sit there for a few minutes, using whatever relaxation techniques help you calm down (e.g., deep breathing, closing your eyes, etc.). Nurses need to give themselves time to relax, refocus, and reenergize.

Positive coping strategies

If ever there was a time to "think nurse," now is the time. Use this mnemonic and its strategies to help you get through your transition period.

Never fail to ask for help. If you don't ask, you may never get help. The best way to get help is to ask for it.

Use available facility resources. You have resources around you—experienced staff, policy and procedure manuals, staff educators, etc. Use them!

Reenergize by joining professional associations. If you were a member of the National Student Nurses Association (NSNA), you already know the benefits of being part of a professional group. There are networking, collegiality, and mentoring opportunities. In addition, being part of your professional organization helps you stay focused on the profession of nursing and why you became a nurse.

Stay in contact with your friends. Everyone needs friends in their busy lives; they are a great resource for relaxation and rejuvenation. Also, stay in touch with your former classmates.

Evaluate your growth realistically. Develop and achieve your short-term goals first and then move on to your long-term goals.

Stay focused on your aspirations. Keep in mind that going through the first year as a nurse is like climbing a hill. It may be hard, but think of how proud you will be when you reach the top (Cherry and Jacob 2005).

Organizational skills

Nurses who have good organizational skills can manage even the worst of days. They always look like they are in control and are never at a loss locating what they need. How do they do it?

Some use a clipboard with a built-in calculator. On this clipboard is also their patient assignment, as well as quick references or "cheat sheets," which are laminated and attached to the back of the board. Others develop a paper worksheet that keeps them on time and organized throughout the shift. Some nurses even use colored markers to organize and prioritize their shifts.

Ask: Talk to your fellow nurses and ask how they organize their workloads. They may have some unique and innovative tips for you to adopt.

Finally, never work in a cluttered environment. Clean your work area before the start of your shift (e.g., your computer on wheels, or medication cart) and always keep your papers in order.

Conflict resolution skills

The best skill to have in your nursing tool belt is conflict resolution. Conflict resolution is the process one uses in resolving a dispute or conflict. Successful conflict resolution occurs when each side's needs and interests are addressed. Each side must also feel good about the outcome. Someone who possesses good conflict-resolution skills can end a potential conflict before it even starts.

Tip: Here are some successful strategies that can help you with conflict resolution:

- Deal with issues that are easiest to resolve first.

- Break the conflict into manageable parts, highlighting where there is common ground.

- Discuss and identify the acceptable and unacceptable aspects of each person's actions and requests.

- Gain agreement in small steps, taking one step at a time.

- Reframe issues in terms of the other person's language or ideology (e.g., "So what you're saying is that you'd like me to listen to your needs more.").

- Demonstrate support and respect for differences.

- Point out the areas of agreement.

- Always maintain a professional demeanor (e.g., low voice, non-abrasive tone, direct eye contact).

- View conflict as a normal, natural process that results from people working together.

References

Austin, S. 2006. "Ladies and gentlemen of the jury, I present . . . the nursing documentation." *Nursing* 36(1): 56–62.

Cherry, B., and S. Jacob. 2005. *Contemporary Nursing Issues, Trends and Management.* St. Louis: Mosby Elsevier.

Kramer, M. 1974. *Reality Shock: Why nurses leave nursing.* St. Louis: Mosby.

Kramer, M., and C. Schalenberg. 1977. *Path to Biculturalism.* Wakefield, MA: Contemporary Publishing, Inc.

Scott, E. 2006. Teaching New Graduate Nurses the Tricks of the Trade. *Tar Heel Nurse* 68(2): 16–17.

Vereb, V. 1981. Reality Shock: Are we coping or copping out? *RN* 44(2): 91–92.

Part Three

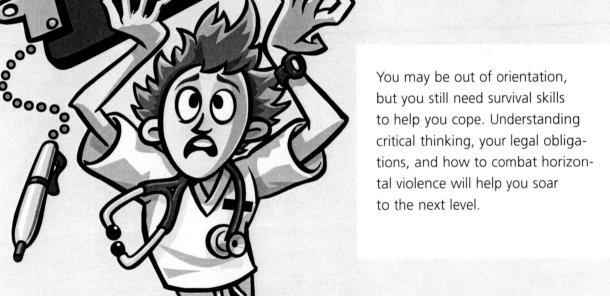

You may be out of orientation, but you still need survival skills to help you cope. Understanding critical thinking, your legal obligations, and how to combat horizontal violence will help you soar to the next level.

Chapter 6

Combating horizontal violence

The scope of the problem

There continues to be a philosophy in the nursing profession that nurses must "earn their stripes." Oftentimes, experienced nurses expect new graduates to put up with harsh treatment and heavy workloads and "sink or swim." Not only does such treatment add further stress to the first-year experience, but it also causes nurses to leave the profession entirely—according to research, approximately 60% of newly registered nurses leave their first position within six months because of some form of horizontal violence (Griffin 2004).

New nurses are initiated into the profession in a variety of negative ways—gossip, bad-mouthing, intimidation, and even bullying. Such behavior is frequently referred to as "nurses eating their young. "You can imagine how destructive this behavior can be during your formative first year.

Watch out: One of the greatest dangers of horizontal violence is that it is insidious and may easily slip under the radar of management. For example, staff nurses may whisper about how a new nurse did not secure an IV "the way it's supposed to be." A fellow nurse may purposefully forget to tell a new nurse about an impromptu staff meeting. A group of nurses may exclude newcomers from joining them at lunch.

> *My floor is notorious for horizontal violence. The day shift is okay, but the 3–11 shift has bickering and the 11–7 shift is just horrible.*
> –2006 Graduate

Unfortunately, such behavior is commonplace and has not changed over the years. Why does it occur, you ask? Well, there are a variety of factors that come into play. First, nurses may feel picked on by physicians and pass those negative feelings on to their colleagues. Second, there may be generational issues at work. More-senior staff nurses may see the younger nurses as over-confident, and resent the fact that they are making top dollar and have no loyalty to the organization. Or, they may feel a new nurse is trying to change the way things are done when "everything is just fine the way it is." Rather than talk these concerns out, nurses express their feelings through disruptive behavior. This inability to communicate and handle conflict is a third factor contributing to the pervasiveness of the problem. We will discuss more theories about why the behavior occurs later in the chapter.

Horizontal violence does not have to plague the nursing profession forever. Together, we must bring the issue into the open and develop a system of open and effective communication. As the newest members of the profession, new graduates like you have a unique opportunity to become "change agents" and improve the culture for the better. So let's get down to business.

What is horizontal violence, exactly?

Fact: Horizontal violence has been defined in nursing literature for more than 20 years and exists under a number of different names and definitions. Here are just a few:

Horizontal violence: "Sabotage directed at coworkers who are on the same level within an organization's hierarchy" (Dunn 2003).

Verbal abuse: "Communication perceived by a person to be a harsh, condemnatory attack, either professional or personal. Language intended to cause distress to a target" (Buback 2004).

Bullying: "The persistent demeaning and downgrading of humans through vicious words and cruel acts that gradually undermine confidence and self-esteem" (Adams 1997).

Horizontal hostility: "A consistent pattern of behavior designed to control, diminish, or devalue a peer (or group) that creates a risk to health and/or safety" (Farrell 2005).

For the sake of clarity, the term "horizontal violence" will be used throughout this chapter.

Horizontal violence is expressed through both covert and overt behaviors and includes any form of mistreatment that leaves a person feeling personally or professionally attacked, devalued, or humiliated (Bartholomew 2006).

Overt examples of horizontal violence include

- name-calling
- bickering
- fault-finding
- backstabbing
- criticism
- intimidation
- gossip
- shouting
- blaming
- using put-downs
- raising eyebrows
- discouragement
- denial of access to opportunities (Bartholomew 2006)

> *I am now getting continuous undermining comments regarding the fact I*
> *pointed out to the unit incomplete assignments I found during my orienta-*
> *tion. Now I get, "Did you do a full assessment (with a laughing undertone)?"*
> *or "You need to stop saying you are sorry during an IV stick—just do it!"*
> **–2006 Graduate, after eight weeks of orientation**

Covert examples of horizontal violence include

- unfair assignments

- sarcasm

- eye-rolling

- ignoring

- making faces behind someone's back

- refusing to help

- sighing/whining

- refusing to work with someone

- sabotage

- isolation

- exclusion

- fabrication (Bartholomew 2006)

Horizontal violence's impact

 Fact: Research focusing on horizontal violence in nursing has been going on for years, with various studies examining both the impact and scope of the problem. A 2003 study published in the *Journal of Advanced Nursing,* for example, looked at nurses' first year of practice and their experiences with horizontal violence. The study found that more than half of the new graduates reported feeling undervalued by other nurses and more than one-third had learning opportunities blocked, experienced overt interpersonal conflict, and/or witnessed behaviors that were rude, abusive, humiliating, or involved unjust criticism. Respondents also reported feeling neglected and distressed by others' conflicts, and cited that they were given too much responsibility without appropriate support (McKenna et al. 2003).

118

Another study published in the *Journal of Advanced Nursing* examined aggression in the clinical setting. The study was conducted to determine

- whether nurses are more concerned about aggression from colleagues than from patients and others

- whether staff-to-staff aggression is common

- whether staff-to-staff aggression is a major cause of work distress for nurses

- what the major forms of aggression among staff are

The study revealed that nurses experienced the most aggression from physicians, followed by patients' relatives, patients, and nurse colleagues. However, the most distressing type of aggression they felt they had to deal with was nurse-to-nurse aggression (Farrell 1999).

Thirty percent of the nurses reported that they experienced aggression on a daily or near-daily basis. The most frequent type of aggression experienced was rudeness, abusive language, humiliation in front of others, and denial of access to opportunities (Farrell 1999).

To deal with the conflict, the most popular action taken by nurses was to talk with a colleague about the experience. The next most common action taken was to speak with the person concerned, a family member, or a manager (Farrell 1999).

Getting to the root of the problem

Here is a quick story to illustrate why horizontal violence exists.

A man was walking by and saw a group of children gathered around a bucket of crabs. One of the crabs was starting to crawl up and out of the bucket. The man said to the children, "you had better put a lid on those crabs, or they'll get out." But to his surprise, the children responded, "Mister, everyone knows you don't need a lid on a bucket of crabs, because every time one tries to get out the other crabs pull it back down" (Bartholomew 2006).

This is a perfect example of why nurses use both blatant and subtle behaviors to demoralize their colleagues. It follows the common mentality: "If I'm miserable here, then everyone else should be too."

There are several theories that explain why horizontal violence exists.

1. **Nursing is an oppressed discipline.** When someone feels inferior, they also feel oppressed. Because there is a strict hierarchy in healthcare, with nursing at the bottom, nurses often feel inferior and powerless. As a result, they take out their tension on their peers. This is clearly a misdirected route for expressing anger.

2. **The demand for efficiency/productivity is too great.** Nurses feel constant pressure to complete their work assignments on time and ensure that nothing is left for the oncoming shift. Because of the heavy workload, there is seldom time to debrief, reflect, and connect with others, which leads to feelings of frustration, depression, and anger. These bottled-up feelings are then released through horizontal violence (Bartholomew 2006).

3. **Nurses suffer from low self-esteem.** The nursing profession is still predominately female. Studies have shown that women have lower self-esteem than men and commonly undervalue their work and themselves. Consequently, nurses with low self-esteem become angry at their own perceived shortcomings, cannot manage their anger appropriately, and attack other nurses (Leiper 2005).

4. **Nurses lack adequate communication and conflict-management skills.** Most nurses prefer to avoid conflict rather than bring it into the open. Having no idea how to confront others and resolve a negative situation, they hide their feelings—or worse, take them out on their innocent coworkers (Bartholomew 2006).

5. **An irrational belief system exists within the nursing profession.** Nurses often hold themselves up to unrealistically high standards (e.g., "I must be perfect and consider myself worthless if I make a mistake," "A good nurse never needs help"). When such beliefs don't match reality, anger results and causes nurses to lash out at one another (Bartholomew 2006).

It is impossible to change the mindset of every nurse in the profession, but we can begin to help make changes in nursing by feeling proud of the work we do and the lives we touch every day.

The consequences of horizontal violence

High levels of interpersonal conflict at work can lead to physical and emotional strain. When you experience horizontal violence, you begin to lose your self-esteem and dread going to work each day.

Watch out: You may see a colleague who experiences such behavior develop fear, anxiety, sadness, and depression. He/she may become frustrated easily and/or mistrust his/her colleagues. Other reported consequences of horizontal violence include post-traumatic stress disorder, increased absenteeism, or leaving the profession of nursing altogether (McKenna et al. 2003).

Fact: Horizontal violence can affect a person in myriad ways. Nurse researcher Gerald Farrell, RN, PhD, cites the following as some of the known effects of verbal abuse:

EMOTIONAL

- Anger, irritability

- Decreased self-esteem

- Lack of motivation and feelings of failure from being unable to meet personal expectations

SOCIAL

- Strained relationships with partner and friends

- Low interpersonal support/absence of emotional support

PSYCHOLOGICAL

- Depression

- Post-traumatic stress disorder (50% continue to suffer from stress five years after the incident)

- Burnout—depersonalization, lack of control

- Maladaptive responses—substance abuse, overeating

PHYSICAL

- Decreased immune response or resistance to infection

- Cardiac arrhythmias (increased risk of heart attack due to continuously circulating catecholamines) (Bartholomew 2006)

The effects of horizontal violence progressively worsen as the behavior continues. William Wilkie, psychiatrist and author of *Understanding Stress Breakdown*, describes the effects of horizontal violence in three stages:

Stage 1: Fight or flight response activated

- Reduced self-esteem

- Sleeping disorders

- Free-floating anxiety

Stage 2: Brain becomes overstimulated and oversensitive

- Difficulty with emotional control—bursting into tears or laughter; irritable and angry

- Difficulty with motivation

Stage 3: Brain's circuit breakers activated

- Intolerance to sensory stimulation

- Loss of ability to ignore things that did not bother you before

- Change in personality (McCarthy et al. 1996)

How do I handle it?

Most nurses like to manage conflict by avoiding it. We like to sweep issues under the rug rather than rock the boat and disturb the status quo. But such an attitude does nothing to solve the problem and improve the work environment.

Don't forget: There are strategies that you can take to avoid becoming a victim of horizontal violence. As a new graduate, you must be willing to ask for help when you need it. And when you have asked for help, always express your appreciation to the nurses who have lent you a hand. Second, do not project an air that you know everything just because you graduated from nursing school. Yes, your opinion is of value, but remember: it is all in your delivery—speaking in a polite and conciliatory tone will get you much more support than being abrasive.

Tip: If you do experience horizontal violence, use open, effective communication to get to the root of the problem. Find someone in a management position who is responsive to ending the behavior and will assist you in putting a stop to the cycle of violence. Discuss the situation with a colleague you trust (or your manger) and role play how you will confront the person(s) involved. That way, you are prepared for the conversation and know how to communicate your side of the situation.

Don't forget: Do not just ignore the behavior, as it will continue or worsen if you allow it to fester. You deserve to be treated as a valued member of the team. If you give respect and consideration, you are entitled to see it in return.

Working with management

If it is apparent that horizontal violence has been going on long before you got there, then it has become an accepted behavior. Make an appointment with your nurse manager or supervisor. Name the problem and use the term "horizontal violence." Stay focused on the behaviors you have observed or experienced. Ask for advice on how best to handle the aggressor. If the response you get is, "She has always been like that. We just ignore it," you need to explain that the behavior is a form of horizontal violence and makes for a hostile work environment. Make every attempt to work with your nurse manager first. If all else fails, go up the chain of command until you get the assistance you need and the behavior changes.

When I was a nurse manager, I encouraged two things. The first was to "send the mail to the right address": I encouraged staff to discuss their interpersonal issues with each other before having me get involved as an intermediary. If they could not resolve the issue on their own, I would sit in as mediator.

Second, I did not allow what Marie Manthey, president of Creative Health Care Management, refers to as the "three Bs" (bitching, bickering, and back-biting). These destructive behaviors can end teamwork and a supportive work environment, which are necessary for nurses to function at their highest level and enjoy the profession they have chosen.

Tip: All nurses, not just new graduates, benefit from education on horizontal violence. Staff members need to know what horizontal violence is, as well as its effects and solutions to its problems. If your unit does not have any education on the topic in place, consider sharing Figure 6.1 with your manager. He/she can then distribute the form to staff or hold an inservice on the subject (Bartholomew 2006).

Figure 6.1: Nurse-to-nurse hostility fact sheet

What is nurse-to-nurse hostility?

Nurse-to-nurse hostility, also known as horizontal violence, colleague abuse, interpersonal conflict among coworkers, and workplace bullying, is a serious issue in the nursing profession that needs to be acknowledged and addressed.

Examples
1. Verbal hostility: Insulting remarks, criticism, bickering, put-downs, shouting, talking behind a colleague's back, name-calling, intimidation, using an inappropriate tone of voice, or withholding information from a colleague regarding a patient.

2. Physical hostility: Turning away, raising eyebrows, refusing to help, ignoring or obstructing the way of a colleague, intimidation using posture, hitting, assaulting, stabbing, or even shooting.

Effects
Feeling of anxiety, fear, shock, anger, and guilt.
Vulnerability, loss of self-confidence, lowered self-esteem, humiliation.
Feeling threatened, developing stress-related illness, and contemplating suicide.

Solutions
At an organizational level:

- Adopt a zero-tolerance policy.

- Embrace transformational leadership (take a stand on issues, inspire, have a positive vision).

- Develop a strong policy to deal with incidents of hostility, including a system of recordkeeping and accountability.

- Develop institutional policies that are proactive, not reactive.

- Develop a workable plan that gives managers the tools to act swiftly when an incident occurs.

- Empower staff to speak without fear of reprisal.

Figure 6.1: Nurse-to-nurse hostility fact sheet (cont.)

At an individual level:

- Gain control. Recognize that the aggressor is at fault—not you.

- Get help from your employer. Read your workplace policy on harassment or horizontal violence to understand your options.

- Make an action plan. Seek advice from others with similar experiences, talk to your manager or counselor, and take advantage of employee assistance programs.

- Take action. Keep a detailed log of all incidents with names of witnesses. If your health is affected by these events, see your healthcare provider.

- Confront the aggressor. Make it clear that the behavior is offensive and must stop. (Use the word "I" and specifically describe the behavior and how it made you feel.)

- Make a formal written complaint. Follow the grievance procedures provided by your organization or union.

- Take legal action. As a last resort, consider seeking expert legal advice.

Source: Jacoba Leiper, RN, MSN, lecturer at the University of North Carolina at Greensboro School of Nursing.

Strategies you can take

If the nursing profession has one flaw, it is a lack of assertiveness. Nurses *must* develop assertiveness skills. Whenever possible, take a class in conflict resolution. Look for a course that will give you concrete skills that you can use in your daily life. An example of a good course would be one that includes practicing effective communication, understanding behavior patterns, recognizing the warning signs, understanding how horizontal violence impacts everyone, and how to prevent it from occurring (Ferns 2006).

In 2004, the *Journal of Continuing Education in Nursing* published a study on the effect of teaching new nurses cognitive skills as a shield from horizontal violence. In the study, the nurses practiced confrontation skills and were given two cards, one listing acceptable behaviors and the other listing appropriate verbal responses to the most common forms of horizontal violence (Figure 6.2). The nurses were able to attach this card to their identification badges so that, in the event of a conflict, they could reference the information immediately (Bartholomew 2006).

Figure 6.2: Cueing cards attached to identification badge

Side 1

Nonverbal innuendo (raising of eyebrows, face-making). I sense (I see from your facial expression) that there may be something you wanted to say to me. It's okay to speak directly to me.

Verbal affront (covert or overt, snide remarks, lack of openness, abrupt responses).
The individuals I learn the most from are clearer in their directions and feedback. Is there some way we can structure this type of situation?

Undermining activities (turning away, being unavailable).
When something happens that is "different" or "contrary" to what I thought or understood, it leaves me with questions. Help me understand how this situation may have happened.

Withholding information (practice or patient).
It is my understanding that there was (is) more information available regarding the situation, and I believe if I had known that (more), it would (will) affect how I learn or need to know.

Sabotage (deliberately setting up a negative situation).
There is more to this situation than meets the eye. Could "you and I" (whatever, whoever) meet in private and explore what happened?

Side 2

Infighting (bickering with peers). Nothing is more unprofessional than a contentious discussion in non-private places. Always avoid. This is not the time or the place. Please stop (physically walk away or move to a neutral spot).

Scapegoating (attributing all that goes wrong to one individual). Rarely is one individual, one incident, or one situation the cause for all that goes wrong. Scapegoating is an easy route to travel, but it rarely solves problems. I don't think that's the right connection.

Backstabbing (complaining to others about an individual and not speaking directly to that individual).
I don't feel right talking about him/her/the situation when I wasn't there or don't know the facts. Have you spoken to him/her?

Failure to respect privacy.
It bothers me to talk about that without his/her/their permission. I only overheard that. It should not be repeated.

Broken confidences.
Wasn't that said in confidence? That sounds like information that should remain confidential. He/she asked me to keep that confidential.

Single card attached to ID

Accept one's fair share of the workload.
Respect the privacy of others.
Be cooperative with regard to the shared physical working conditions (e.g., light, temperature, noise).
Be willing to help when requested.
Keep confidences.
Work cooperatively despite feelings of dislike.
Don't denigrate to superiors (e.g., speak negatively about, have a pet name for).
Do address coworkers by their first name, and ask for help and advice when necessary.
Look coworkers in the eye when having a conversation.
Don't be overly inquisitive about each others' lives.
Do repay debts, favors, and compliments, no matter how small.
Don't engage in conversation about a coworker with another coworker.
Stand up for the "absent member" in a conversation when he/she is not present.
Don't criticize publicly.

Source: SLACK Incorporated and The Journal of Continuing Education in Nursing. *Reprinted with permission*

Chapter 7

A guide to
critical thinking

The uninquiring life is not the life for man.
                                    –Socrates

Learning how to think like a nurse: Head versus hands

When you were in the clinical setting, whether in a simulated lab or at the hospital, you were asked many questions by your instructor and the staff with whom you worked. These questions were designed to make you begin to "think" like a nurse versus "acting" like a nurse. The world of healthcare today desperately needs professionals who are critical thinkers, and not robots that simply do tasks.

Fact: Developing critical thinking in nursing students has become a major initiative in nursing education and is cited as a desirable outcome in most professional education programs. The National League for Nursing Accrediting Commission criteria No. 13A cited critical thinking as an essential skill for nursing curricula. The Commission on Collegiate Nursing Education identifies critical thinking as a core competency in baccalaureate nursing education. The term "critical thinking" frequently appears in various education and nursing journals.

Like many skills, however, critical thinking takes time to develop; while all nurses have the *ability* to think critically, it is not a skill that comes effortlessly—especially for new graduates. In a 2005 study published in *Nursing Education Perspectives*, only 35% of new RN graduates studied—regardless of educational preparation—met the entry expectations for clinical judgment. The study concluded that employers cannot expect new RN graduates to be completely competent; however, they can expect that the new graduate meet safe-entry expectations (Del Bueno 2005).

As a new graduate, you need to get on the path toward critical thinking immediately. The sooner you develop your skills in this area, the sooner you will be able to practice soundly and reduce your chances of making poor patient-care decisions. This chapter will help you understand what critical thinking is, the characteristics of a critical thinker, and strategies to help you cultivate these qualities in yourself and in practice.

The roots of critical thinking

Theories of critical thinking can be traced back to the Greek philosophers. Socrates believed that all traditions and assumptions were open to critical examination. Plato, a student of Socrates, believed that education should provide not only information, but also aim to allow students to question, examine, and reflect upon ideas and values. Aristotle asserted that critical thinking combined abstract thinking and logical thinking.

In the 20th century, philosopher and psychologist John Dewey explored "reflective thinking" in his book *How We Think* and suggested that critical thinking was a subset of the reflective process, involving thorough assessment, scrutiny, and the drawing of conclusions in relation to the issue at hand (Daly 1998).

More recently, Michael Scriven and Richard Paul, in a statement for the National Council for Excellence in Critical Thinking Instruction, described critical thinking as an intellectually disciplined process that is

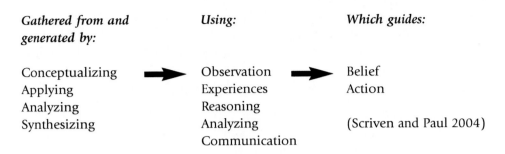

Gathered from and generated by:		*Using:*		*Which guides:*
Conceptualizing		Observation		Belief
Applying		Experiences		Action
Analyzing		Reasoning		
Synthesizing		Analyzing		(Scriven and Paul 2004)
		Communication		

Scriven and Paul defined critical thinking as having two components "1) a set of information and belief-generating and processing skills, and 2) the habit, based on intellectual commitment, of using those skills to guide behavior. It is thus to be contrasted with 1) the mere acquisition and retention of information alone, because it involves a particular way in which information is sought and treated; 2) the mere possession of a set of skills, because it involves the continual use of them; and 3) the mere use of those skills ('as an exercise') without acceptance of their results" (Scriven and Paul 2004).

Definitions of critical thinking

There are many definitions of critical thinking. Here are a few of the most widely accepted:

- "Thinking that is purposeful, reasoned, and goal directed" (Halpern 1989)

- "A composite of attitudes, knowledge, and skills that include attitudes of inquiry that involve an ability to recognize the existence of problems and an acceptance of the general need for evidence in support of what is asserted to be true; knowledge of the nature of valid abstractions and generalizations in which the weight or accuracy of different kinds of evidence is logically determined; skills in employing and applying the above attitudes and knowledge" (Watson and Glaser 1991)

- "A mode of thinking—about any subject, content, or problem—in which the thinker improves the quality of his or her thinking by skillfully taking charge of the structures inherent in thinking and imposing intellectual standards about them" (Scriven and Paul 2004)

What we can take away from all of these definitions is that a nurse with critical thinking skills is a well-rounded person who possesses the capacity to think with given variables and has the ability to weigh these variables to achieve a good patient outcome.

Critical thinking versus problem-solving

Don't forget: While there are many definitions of critical thinking, the term should not be confused with decision-making, problem-solving, or clinical judgment. Each is a separate set of skills necessary in becoming a good nurse.

Problem-solving is far different from critical thinking. In fact, problem-solving conflicts with the process orientation of critical thinking. Remember that critical thinking is an outcome-oriented thinking that is based on scientific knowledge and evidence-based practice. Problem-solving is merely seeking a single solution to a problem and consists of the following four key components:

1. Identifying assumptions
2. Challenging assumptions
3. Recognizing the context of the problem
4. Exploring alternatives (Boychuk Duchscher 1999)

Clinical judgment, on the other hand, **is** rooted in the critical thinking process. Catherine Tanner defined clinical judgment as a series of decisions made by the nurse when dealing with the patient, regarding

- observations made in the patient situation

- evaluation of the data observed and formulation of meaning (diagnosis)

- nursing actions that should be taken on behalf of the patient (Tanner 1987)

Tanner's definition looks a lot like the nursing process. In school, you learned that the *nursing process* is a scientific approach to providing patient care. Its objective is to provide a rational approach to problem solving. The goal of the nursing process—and critical thinking—is to uncover the best solution by applying a complete set of steps.

Characteristics of critical thinkers

> *We are what we repeatedly do. Excellence, then, is not an act, but a habit.*
> –Aristotle

The American Philosophical Association defines the ideal critical thinker as being "habitually inquisitive, well-informed, trustful of reason, open-minded, flexible, fair-minded in evaluation, honest in facing personal biases, prudent in making judgments, willing to reconsider, clear about issues, orderly in complex matters, diligent in seeking relevant information, reasonable in selection of criteria, focused in inquiry, and persistent in seeking results which are as precise as the subject and the circumstances of the inquiry permit" (American Philosophical Association 1990).

Stephen Brookfield, author of *Developing Critical Thinkers: Challenging Adults to Explore Alternative Ways of Thinking and Acting*, characterized critical thinkers as people who engage in productive and positive activity, and see their thinking as a process rather than an outcome. They vary in their manifestations of critical thinking according to the circumstance and feel comfortable with the emotional as well as the rational elements of the critical thinking process (Brookfield 1991).

Figure 7.1: Attributes of a critical thinker

- Asks pertinent questions
- Assesses statements and arguments
- Is curious about things
- Listens to others and is able to give feedback
- Looks for evidence or proof
- Examines problems closely
- Can reject information that is not relevant or is incorrect
- Wants to find the solution

- Thinks independently
- Questions deeply
- Maintains intellectual integrity
- Confident in rationale for actions
- Analyzes arguments
- Evaluates evidence and facts
- Explores consequences before taking action
- Recognizes a contradiction
- Evaluates policy

Source: Ferrett, S. 1997. Peak Performance: Success in College and Beyond. *New York: McGraw-Hill.*

Critical thinking in nursing

> *The characteristic that distinguishes a professional nurse*
> *is cognitive rather than psychomotor ability.*
> –Kataoka-Yahiro and Saylor

Fact: The reason critical thinking is so important in nursing is based on what nursing does as a profession. Because we deal with people, there is much we must take into consideration and there are direct consequences to our nursing actions. Just think about what nurses are facing today. The practice of nursing is done in the face of multiple and competing pathologies. Each patient is unique in their physical structure and their personal needs based on social, gender, cultural, and/or religious norms. Nurses also have to take into consideration the patient's cognitive abilities and the availability of the patient's human and non-human resources. There is never a "one-size-fits-all" solution to providing care.

Critical thinking is vital because it directs us in providing safe, competent care. Nurses who possess critical thinking skills make a difference in decreasing hospital stays and producing good patient outcomes. Again, the nurse who uses his/her "head" versus just his/her "hands" is of value to any organization.

Learning the art of critical thinking

Ask: For you to become a critical thinker you must first answer the following questions. Be honest in your evaluation.

- What have you learned about how you think?

- What do you know about how to analyze, evaluate, or reconstruct your thinking?

- Where does your thinking come from? How much of it is based on past modes of thinking versus new, "out-of-the-box" thinking?

- How much of your thinking is vague, muddled, inaccurate, illogical, or superficial?

- Have you ever discovered a problem in your thinking and then changed it (Elder 2002)?

Given our fast-paced society, you would not be alone if you could not answer these questions. Most colleges do not offer courses on the topic of "thinking" and we live in a culture that shows very little interest in furthering our cognitive skills. But there are ways to become better at thinking. Just like a professional baseball player, musician, or artist, you will need to practice.

Tip: Here are some strategies for you to use to improve your critical thinking:

- **Clarify your thinking.** Summarize in your own words what others have said.

- **Stick to the point.** Look out for fragmented thinking, or thinking that leaps about with no logical connection.

- **Value questions.** Listen to how your patients ask questions, when they ask questions, and when they do not ask questions. You must also ask questions in order to understand and effectively deal with your environment. A well-cultivated critical thinker in nursing is able to both raise vital questions and formulate them clearly.

- **Be reasonable and open-minded.** One of the characteristics of a critical thinker is the ability to change one's mind when given good reason to change. Do you become irritated by the reasons someone gives or do you become defensive during a discussion? Can you be moved by reason or are you unwilling to listen to others' reasons? (Elder and Paul 2002)

- **Gather and assess relevant information.** Once you have done this, use abstract ideas to interpret the information and reach well-reasoned conclusions. In addition, test the solutions against relevant criteria and standards.

- **Communicate effectively with others.** One of the best ways to find a solution to a complex patient problem is to consult your experienced colleagues.

The six skills of an expert thinker

According to a 2001 article in *Dimensions of Critical Care Nursing*, there are six essential cognitive skills that a nurse needs to be considered an expert critical thinker:

1. **Interpretation.** This skill involves clarifying meaning. You need to be able to interpret subjective and objective data. Do you understand the significance of lab values, vital signs, and physical assessment data?

2. **Analysis.** Based on your assessment data, can you analyze and determine the patient's problem is?

3. **Evaluation.** This involves the identification of expected patient outcomes and assessing whether or not they were met. If they were not met, can you determine why?

4. **Inference,** which is the act of drawing conclusions (e.g., based on careful monitoring, you determine whether a patient's health status is improving or declining).

5. **Explanation,** or the nurse's ability to justify actions. This is based on the nurse using research or other sources of evidence when doing nursing interventions.

6. **Self-regulation,** which is the process of looking at your own practice and correcting or improving it (Ignatavicius 2001).

Testing one, two, three

During your orientation program, you may be "tested" on how well you can think critically. Hospitals use various methods to accomplish this, including simulation labs and the Performance Based Development System (PBDS).

A simulation lab will test your skills and use of standards. This can be done during a mock code, for example, where you may be asked

- Do you know the principles of the AHA (American Heart Association) standards?

- Can you figure out what to do when things don't go as planned (or taught)?

- What did you learn from the simulated experience?

- What would you do differently next time?

The second testing method, PBDS, relies on a competency-assessment system that has been around since the 1980s. Under this system, three areas of performance are assessed: critical thinking skills, interpersonal skills, and technical skills. Evaluators look for you to display specific qualities within each area.

1. **Critical thinking** (doing the right thing for the right reason)

    - Problem recognition
    - Risk and problem management
    - Priority setting
    - Application of knowledge

2. **Interpersonal skills** (how well do you get along with people)

    - Conflict resolution
    - Customer satisfaction
    - Team building

3. **Technical skills** (doing the right thing)

    - Safe performance of procedures
    - Effective use of equipment
    - Efficient use of time and resources

The PBDS system uses three patient-focused exercises that are tested at three different levels of difficulty. The simplest exercise uses a variety of written patient events to evaluate your ability to determine which patient is your priority and how you manage that patient. The second exercise is visual and out of context. It is used to evaluate how you would recognize and manage peripheral IV problems as well as aseptic technique. The third, most complex exercise consists of patient video simulations that evaluate your ability to

- accurately identify any patient problems

- safely manage those problems in an appropriate timeframe

- support your nursing actions with appropriate rationales
  (Del Bueno 2005)

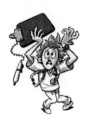

Don't panic: What if you do not do well in this type of testing? Any nurse with an unacceptable assessment should plan more clinical practice and develop an evaluation plan with his/her preceptor or manager. Remember, you are a novice nurse with problem-solving abilities, using clinical judgment to make patient-care decisions. You just need time and practice in moving from problem-solving to critical thinking.

Final thoughts

Critical thinking is never constant in any individual, no matter what his/her experience level. Everyone has episodes of undisciplined or irrational thought. Just think about what happens in times of stress. We begin to lose focus, have self-doubt, and take the path of least resistance. To become a nurse with good critical thinking skills, you must commit to the development of critical thinking as a life long undertaking. Be a critic of your own thinking and you'll soon begin reaping the benefits of improved outcomes and patient care.

References

American Association of Colleges of Nursing. 1998. *The Essentials of Baccalaureate Education for Professional Nursing Practice.*

American Philosophical Association. 1990. *Critical Thinking: A Statement of Expert Consensus for Purposes of Educational Assessment and Instruction.* Millbrae, CA: The California Academic Press.

Boychuck Duchscher, J. 1999. Catching the wave: Understanding the concept of critical thinking. *Journal of Advanced Nursing* 29(3): 577–583.

Brookfield, S. 1991. *Developing Critical Thinkers: Challenging Adults to Explore Alternative Ways of Thinking and Acting.* San Francisco: Jossey-Bass/Wiley.

Daly, W. 1998. Critical thinking as an outcome of nursing education. What is it? Why is it important to nursing practice? *Journal of Advanced Nursing* 28(2): 323–31.

Del Bueno, D. 2005. Crisis in Critical Thinking. *Nursing Education Perspectives* 26(5): 278–282.

Elder, L., and Paul, R. 2002. *Becoming a Critic of Your Thinking: Tools for Taking Charge of Your Professional and Personal Life.* Upper Saddle River, New Jersey: Financial Times/Prentice Hall.

Facione, N., and P. Facione. 1994. *Holistic Critical Thinking Scoring Rubric.* Millbrae, CA: The California Academic Press.

Ferrett, S. 1997. *Peak Performance: Success in College and Beyond.* New York: McGraw-Hill.

Halpern, D. 1989. *Thought and Knowledge: An Introduction to Critical Thinking,* 2nd ed. NJ: Lawrence Erlbaum Associates.

Ignatavicius, D. 2001. Six critical thinking skills for at-the-bedside success. *Dimensions of Critical Care Nursing* 20(2): 30–33.

Katoaka-Yahiro, M., and C. Saylor. 1994. A critical thinking model for nursing judgment. *Journal of Nursing Education* 33(8): 351–356

National League for Nursing Accrediting Commission, Inc. 2004. *Accreditation Manual with Interpretative Guidelines by Program Type. www.nlnac.org/*

Schank, M. 1990. Wanted: Nurses with critical thinking skills. *The Journal of Continuing Education in Nursing* 21(2): 86–89.

Scriven, M., and R. Paul. Defining Critical Thinking: A statement for the National Council for Excellence in Critical Thinking Instruction. *www.criticalthinking.org.*

Tanner, C. 1987. Teaching clinical judgment. *Annual Review of Nursing Research* 5: 153–173.

Turner, P. 2005. Critical Thinking in Nursing Education and Practice as Defined in the Literature. *Nursing Education Perspectives* 26(5): 272–277.

Watson, G., and E. Glaser. 1991. *Critical Thinking Appraisal Manual.* Kent, England: Psychological Corporation.

Chapter 8

New-nurse survival skills

When you were in nursing school, you probably could not wait until graduation. No more cramming for exams, writing papers, or worrying about passing your tests. Now that you've entered the nursing profession, however, you've undoubtedly encountered a whole new set of stressors—starting a new job, adjusting to a demanding schedule, cultivating collegial relationships with everyone on staff, etc. While these events may seem scary, there are strategic "survival" skills that you can develop to face stress, improve your communication style, and resolve conflict. This chapter will cover each of those skills so that you are more than prepared for your first year—and beyond.

Survival skill #1: Stress management

Stress is the #1 health problem in America, and job stress is the major culprit. Nursing can be a stressful profession, especially depending on where you work and how you handle stress in your daily life.

Ask: People become stressed and burned out because they think that they have little control over their environment and their future. Do not fall into this trap! **Focus on what you can control** and you will realize that there are many things you can do to improve your environment.

When you learn how to manage your stress, it allows you to experience life from a more positive perspective. In fact, studies have shown that when we view stress as a positive rather than negative experience, it leads us to happier and more fulfilled lives.

How stressed are you?

Before we delve into skills for handling stress, take the following test to determine the level of work and personal stress you are currently facing. To calculate your total stress points, add up those life events you have experienced in the past year.

Figure 8.1: Life event stress test

Life event		Points	Life event		Points	Life event		Points
Death of a spouse or partner	❑	100	Significant change to financial status	❑	37	Trouble with employer	❑	23
Divorce	❑	73	Death of a close friend	❑	36	Change in working hours or conditions	❑	20
Marital separation	❑	65	Change in line of work	❑	35	Moving house	❑	20
Serving a jail sentence	❑	63	Increase in domestic arguments	❑	35	Changing school	❑	20
Death of a close relative	❑	63	Large mortgage	❑	31	Change in recreation	❑	20
Serious illness or injury	❑	53	Foreclosure of mortgage or loan	❑	30	Change in church activities	❑	19
Marriage	❑	50	More or less responsibility at work	❑	29	Change in social life	❑	19
Loss of job	❑	47	Child leaving home	❑	29	Taking out a small mortgage	❑	17
Marital reconciliation	❑	45	Friction with in-laws	❑	29	Sleep problems	❑	16
Retirement	❑	45	Outstanding personal achievement	❑	28	Change in family get-togethers	❑	15
Change in family member's health	❑	44	Spouse starting or ending work	❑	26	Change in eating habits	❑	15
Pregnancy	❑	40	Starting or completing education	❑	26	Going on vacation	❑	13
Sexual difficulties	❑	39	Change in living conditions	❑	25	Christmas	❑	12
New baby or family member	❑	39	Change in personal habits	❑	24	Minor violation of the law	❑	11

Your overall score: _____

Source: Gill, Jit. 2003. Stress Survival Guide. NY: HarperTorch.

If your total score for this activity is less than 150 points, you have a low susceptibility to developing a stress-related illness. If, however, you scored more than 150 points, you have a 50% chance of developing a stress-related illness in the near future. If you scored more than 300 points, you have a 90% chance of developing a stress-related illness in the near future. Anyone with a score of 150 or more should learn and practice stress management.

Types of stress

By identifying where your stress originates, you will be able to better take control of the pressures surrounding you. Stress comes in a variety of forms and from a number of places. The following are the most common types:

- **Personal stress.** Comes from your personal life and includes your own perception of yourself and relationships. Impacts your self-esteem and feelings of self-worth.

- **Physiological stress.** Results from various kinds of stress and how your body responds to the stress.

- **Social stress.** Related to your perceived appearance in the world. For example, the personal stressor of getting married is also a source of social stress. Why? Because there will be societal opinions and reactions to your new marital relationship.

- **Environmental stress.** Largely unavoidable stress caused by the nature of the world around us (e.g., noise and visual stimuli).

Symptoms of stress

Our bodies react to stress in a number of negative ways. Stress affects our mental and emotional states by making us feel angry, jealous, fearful, anxious, and/or depressed. It lowers our self-esteem and our ability to concentrate and make decisions. Stress manifests itself physically through muscular aches and pains, poor posture, puffy eyes and dehydrated skin (Gill 1999).

When the body is overloaded with too much stress, burnout results. We see burnout in nursing because nurses do not recognize the signs and symptoms of stress in themselves, or do not take care of themselves to avoid burnout. In fact, burnout in our profession has become so common that 40% of hospital nurses have burnout levels that exceed the norms for healthcare workers (Aiken et. al 2002).

Be on the lookout for signs of burnout, which include loss of motivation, interest, and energy; emotional exhaustion; no longer wanting to be around work or family; disillusionment; persistent feelings of frustration; and a loss of interest in personal hygiene (Adamson 2002).

Coping with stress

Your ability to cope with stress is dependent upon how well you can deal with the demands of everyday life. You probably know people who feel they are at the mercy of uncontrollable, unforeseen demands—they are the ones with poor coping skills. People with strong coping skills, however, deal well with anything that comes their way and have learned to be assertive, think rationally, stay organized in their work and home lives, have quality relationships, and take care of themselves properly. Are you taking notes? All of those life skills will help you cope with the stressors of being a nurse.

When you notice that you are bothered by the stressors of life, Adamson suggests practicing some of the following techniques. The x's indicate which type of stress the technique most effectively addresses.

Figure 8.2: Coping techniques

Technique	Type of stress			
	Personal	Physiological	Social	Environmental
Attitude adjustment			X	
Ayurveda (form of alternative medicine dealing with healthy living and therapeutic, holistic measures)		X		
Breathing exercises				X
Creative therapy	X		X	X
Dream journaling	X			
Exercise	X	X	X	X
Feng shui				X
Friend therapy	X		X	
Habit reshaping	X	X	X	
Meditation	X	X		
Massage therapy	X	X		
Nutrition		X		X
Optimism therapy	X			
Relaxation techniques	X	X		
Self-hypnosis	X			
Visualization	X	X	X	
Vitamin/mineral therapy, herbal medicine, homeopathy		X		X

Source: Adamson, E. 2002. The Everything Stress Management Book: Practical ways to relax, be healthy, and maintain your sanity. Avon, MA: Adams Media.

Keep in mind that there is no single coping method that is uniformly successful. Just because your friend finds that jogging works for him does not mean that it will work for you. Only you can decide what works best for your lifestyle and goals. For example, if trying to get to the health club before or after work only causes you more stress, drop it and explore another method. Find an exercise that you like to do and can do on your own time, like walking or yoga.

Additional methods for overcoming stress

Cognitive-behavioral techniques
Cognitive-behavioral methods are very effective in stress reduction and rely on identifying sources of stress, restructuring priorities, discussing your feelings, looking for the positive, and using humor.

Identifying sources of stress

Ask: Tackle stress head-on by first determining where your stress originates. Keep a log of your daily events with the date and time of the activities and any key words to point out how you felt. Now see if you can pinpoint which events caused you stress. When did you become tired, angry, or feel anxious? Did you develop any physical ailment, such as a headache? Also be sure to include those things which made you feel good during the day, as these activities may alert you to what coping techniques work best for you.

This exercise should help you identify the sources of stress so that you can now develop a plan for how to control or minimize it.

Restructuring priorities
Restructuring your priorities will help you shift the balance from stress-producing to stress-reducing activities. You will never be able to completely eliminate stress from your life, but you can control and reduce it by striking a balance between work and fun.

Think about what activities make you happy and try to build them into your schedule. Examples include taking a long weekend, planning a special vacation each year, taking a break from a stressful work or home environment (even if it is only for one hour), and making time for things you enjoy, such as recreational activities or hanging out with friends.

Discussing your feelings

This is a great way to reduce stress. The worst thing you can do is to keep your feelings of anger or frustration to yourself. Not discussing your feelings with a friend, colleague, or family member can lead to hostility, feelings of helplessness, and even depression. If talking to others is not a comfortable option for you, try writing your feelings in a journal or letter.

Looking for the positive

This is a way to reverse negative ideas and feelings. Train yourself to focus on the positive (e.g., seeing the glass as half full rather than half empty). If you can learn to focus on positive outcomes, you will help yourself reduce tension and accomplish your goals.

Using humor

This technique is one of my favorites. Everyone knows that humor has therapeutic effects on the body. It helps us cope with stress and difficult situations. Just think about your own world of friends and family. Doesn't everyone like being around the funny guy? Yes, and that's because such people help us laugh at life and ourselves.

It will be hard for you to find humor in your first year, but when you do find it, you'll know you have arrived as a nurse, because you are no long taking yourself and others so seriously (American Institute of Stress 2006).

The importance of a healthy lifestyle

Following a healthy lifestyle keeps your body and mind in top-notch condition so that when stress comes your way, you are mentally and physically prepared to handle it. If you are not already pursuing a healthy lifestyle, now is the time to start. You will be thankful you did a few years down the road.

Click: Healthy living starts with a healthy diet. Go to *www.mypyramid.gov*. There, you will see a box that asks you for your age, gender, and activity level. Once you have submitted the information, a diet plan will appear that includes your portions for grains, vegetables, fruits, milk, meat, and beans. Follow this plan and you will start off on the right foot. Also be sure you are getting enough adequate vitamins and minerals. Do not skip any meals and avoid ingredients that worsen the negative effects of stress on your body, such as caffeine, sugar, fat, salt, and extra calories.

Part of a healthy lifestyle also includes exercise. Exercise is a great way to clear your head of everyday stressors. It doesn't mean you have to join a health club, per se. Find an activity you like to do and mark it on the calendar—it's like making an appointment with yourself. Start out by exercising once a week (if you don't typically exercise) and gradually increase to at least three times per week. Many times I see my neighbors start out with good intentions in the spring by jogging. Within less than one month I no longer see them jogging. I often wonder why they didn't start out small, like walking first to build up their stamina. Whatever you plan for yourself, take it in small steps and build on those successes.

Stress-proofing work

You will find nursing a rewarding profession, but it does have its sources of stress. The key is to get this stress under control from day one. Start out by identifying what areas of your work are causing you the most stress. Is it something you can change? If so, develop a plan and put it into action.

Tip: There are various ways you can manage on-the-job stressors, such as

- avoiding the stressor (e.g., a nurse who is rude to you)

- eliminating the stressor (e.g., asking someone else to do a hated chore for you)

- confronting the stressor (e.g., talking with the person(s) who are making your job more difficult)

- managing the stressor (e.g., adding something fun to the task, or better yet, rewarding yourself once it's done)

- balancing the stressor (e.g., balancing it with a stress-reducing technique) (Adamson 2002)

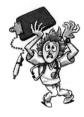

Don't panic: If you really believe you have tried all of the appropriate avenues to help relieve job stress, but it still exists, then you need to think about changing jobs. There are plenty of positions out there that will meet your expectations and cause you less stress.

Stress-proofing your home

You will now have to divide your precious time between work and home. The everyday demands of grocery shopping, cleaning, paying bills and running errands will take up your time and cause you stress if you do not learn how to manage them well.

Tip: Consider following some of these stress busters:

- Hire outside help for your weekly or every-other-week cleaning.

- Always put things back where you found them and teach others who live with you to do the same.

- Declutter your life. When you buy something new, throw out something old.

- Make a list of chores for the outside and inside of the house; divide them up with everyone who lives there.

- Keep a record of all of your expenses. After 3–6 months, review it and set up a reasonable budget that you can live by.

- Have your paycheck directly deposited into your bank account. This will save you time at the bank.

- Pay your bills online. You can even set it up to pay certain bills automatically each month.

Stress-proofing for life

Only you can determine what stress management techniques work best for you. Even finding one thing that will assist you with coping with the stressors of life will be of benefit.

Consider changing the bad habits that increase your stress and concentrate on some new everyday things that can help you stay in control. These things could be as simple as setting your alarm on your cell phone to remind you of appointments, taking a few deep relaxing breaths, staying away from working lunches, using your commute as a time to relax and listen to soothing music, teaching the kids to give you five minutes in the house before they start demanding your time, planning a mental health day (day off from work) at least once every three months, and developing a sense of humor and learning to have fun!

Tip: Here are some final stress busters you can practice:

- Be kind to yourself and keep your expectations realistic. You have a lifetime in nursing—you don't have to do it all in the first year.

- Watch people who seem to "have their act together." Ask them how they do it.

- For those of us who cannot sit still for the quieter forms of relaxation techniques, use more active forms of stress management, such as strenuous exercise and yard work.

- Focus on small escapes, like a 10-minute walk outside or a long weekend, rather than a big vacation.

- Stop by the newborn nursery. Who wouldn't be happy after seeing a new life?

- Get some outdoor time everyday.

- Laugh every day at the absurd.

- Develop friends outside of nursing; they may have interesting insights for you.

- Limit fast food unless it's healthy fast food.

- Everyone benefits from some kind of mind-quieting activity; take a few minutes of peace and quiet in the middle of your busy day. It can do wonders.

- Never let anyone abuse you—not patients, bosses, peers, or friends.

- Lose high-maintenance people (unless you are married to them or were born to them).

- Make music and flowers part of your everyday life.

- Try being just a little bit organized—it will do wonders for your stress level.

- Stay away from negative people; they will just drag you down with them.

- Make sure you have a personal life.

- Set boundaries between work and home.

- Be a good steward of your time, talents, energy, efforts, and resources.

- Be your own cheerleader.

Survival skill #2: Effective communication

Communication is a complex exchange of information through verbal and non-verbal means. It starts as soon as two or more people become aware of each other's presence.

Click: If you are unsure of your communication style, visit *www.queendom.com/tests/relationships/communication_skills_r_access.html*, where you can take a 34-question test to determine your level of interpersonal communication skills.

Communication inventory

Ask: To determine if you are practicing effective communication skills, ask yourself these questions:

- Am I open to the opinions and expertise of others?

- Am I capable of communicating without judgment?

- Do I have strong listening skills?

- Am I capable of expressing empathy to clients and colleagues?

If you are honestly doing these things, give yourself a pat on the back—you are well on your way! If not, don't panic. Developing effective communication skills is not difficult—with a little diligence, you can improve this skill in no time.

The components of communication

To become an effective communicator, you must be able to use nonverbal and verbal communication and listening skills.

Figure 8.3: Sender-message-receiver model of communication

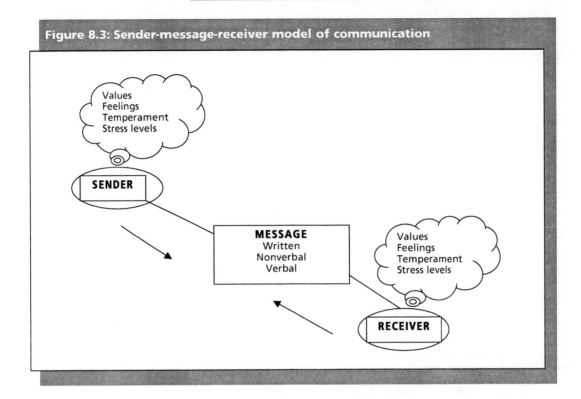

Nonverbal skills

When examining your nonverbal skills, remember that space, environment, appearance, eye contact, posture, gestures, facial expressions, timing, tone, volume, and inflection will all be interpreted by the receiver. Note your position when having a conversation—are you facing the speaker and making eye contact? Be sensitive to the cues you are sending, as well those you are receiving.

Fact: Communication is typically 7% verbal, 38% vocal, and 55% visual, so you can see how body language plays a major role in how your message is heard. You are sending poor signals when you fold your arms, roll your eyes, do not have eye contact, do something else, lean back, or allow for interruptions. Remember that when the nonverbal and verbal messages do not match (e.g., you say you are listening but are looking in another direction), the receiver is more likely to believe the nonverbal message. Our bodies give hidden messages all of the time, so be careful in your nonverbal communication.

Tip: To become an effective communicator you will have to learn how to use your body language in a positive way:

- Smile

- Make eye contact

- Acknowledge with head nodding

- Give a firm handshake

- Touch the other person's hand, forearm, or upper back

- Maintain appropriate "personal space"

- Sit or stand face to face

- Sit or lean forward

- Use silence appropriately

Verbal skills

Verbal communication takes into account your tone and inflection. The receiver is listening to your words and the emphasis placed on specific words in the message. Look at this simple sentence and say each one with the emphasis on the italicized word:

- You are going to *pay* for this.

- *You* are going to pay for this.

- You *are going* to pay for this.

Each sentence conveys a different meaning. The first sentence gives the impression that it could be a question. In the second, you may think that only "you" are going to pay and no one else. The last sentence gives the impression of anger. This exercise should make it clear that the way in which you say a message can be misunderstood if you do not pay careful attention (Cherry 2005).

Listening skills

Listening skills are a major part of effective communication. When speaking with others "actively listen" and look for both the verbal and nonverbal cues. There are so many distractions in nursing that you really have to learn how to listen effectively to your patients, families, peers, and physicians.

See how many essential effective listening skills you have:

_____ I can hear what is being said (no distractions and I do not talk).

_____ I focus my attention on what is being said, not doing two things at once.

_____ I can control my emotions despite what is being said.

_____ I decide right in the beginning to listen and accept the other person's needs and feelings.

_____ I pay attention to nonverbal communication as I am listening to the words.

_____ I take notes when there is a lot of factual information being shared.

_____ I allow the speaker to tell the whole story.

_____ I react to the message and not the person delivering the message

(Zerwekh and Claborn 2006)

Don't forget: If you are in a noisy area, take the conversation to a quieter location. Do not be afraid to politely interrupt the speaker and ask for clarification if you do not understand his/her message. Use rephrasing to be sure you understand the intended message. When you use active listening skills, you are sending the message that the other person is of value, you have an interest in what he/she has to say, and you care enough to listen.

Basic principles of effective communication

1. You are responsible for making sure your message is clear.

2. Use the KISS (Keep It Short and Simple) principle.

3. Match your nonverbal and verbal behaviors so that there is no misinterpretation.

4. Always "send the message to the right address." Speak with the person directly and not around them.

5. Keep your biases in check. Do not let them interfere with your communication and message.

6.   Always be respectful of the other person.

7.   Never lower yourself down a level. If the other person is yelling or attempting to degrade you, don't go there. You always come out a winner when you maintain your integrity.

Survival skill #3: Conflict resolution

Do not wait for leaders; do it alone, person to person.
–Mother Teresa

Just like stress, there is no way to avoid conflict in our lives. It is a normal process of life. The causes of conflict stem from problems with communication, differences in what each person wants from a given situation, differences in how to get to an agreed outcome, and personality differences.

Conflict resolution is the process of resolving a dispute or conflict. Successful conflict resolution occurs when each side's needs and interests are addressed in such a way that each side is satisfied with the outcome.

Ways of handling conflict

There are five common ways of dealing with conflict. Not all are effective or healthy, but it's important that you understand each so that are prepared to handle any situation that comes your way.

Figure 8.4: Ways of dealing with conflict

Method	Result
Denial or withdrawal	You attempt to get rid of conflict by denying that it exists. The conflict will not go away and it will grow to the point that it becomes unmanageable. If the issue is not critical, denial may be appropriate.
Suppression or smoothing over	When suppression is used, it plays down differences and does not recognize the positive aspects of handling the conflict openly. The source of the conflict seldom goes away. The only time suppression should be used is when the issue is relatively insignificant and you are trying to preserve the relationship.
Power or dominance	Power is often used to settle differences. But power strategies result in winners and losers—and the losers will not support the final decision in the same way as the winners.
Compromise or negotiation	This solution may be weakened to the point that it will not be accepted. There may be little real commitment by any of the persons involved. Compromise works when the resources are limited and a speedy decision needs to be made.
Integration or collaboration	All persons involved recognize the interests of the other. Each person's interests, positive intentions, and desired outcomes are explored. Each person's views are adapted as the work progresses. There is recognition of value in what each person brings to the discussion.

Source: Oregon Mediation Center, Inc. 2006. Effective mediation resources: Training Manual. www.internetmediator.com/medres/.

Managing conflict

Watch out: Responding to conflict is a skill that you must have in today's workplace. You need to be able to stay calm and keep the communication lines open. During a conflict you need to avoid emotional triggers:

- Criticism: "You brought this on yourself."

- Preaching: "You should think of others before you act."

- Advising: "If I were you I'd . . ."

- Side tracking: "If you think that was bad, let me tell you about . . . "

(SkillPath 1995)

The following strategies can contribute to positive conflict resolution:

- Deal with safer issues first.

- Break the conflict into manageable parts and highlight where there is common ground. Emphasize points of consensus.

- Identify the acceptable and unacceptable aspects of each alternative suggested.

- Gain consensus one step at a time.

- Demonstrate support and respect for differences; build a culture of tolerance.

- Separate the person from the issue.

- Maintain a professional demeanor.

- Do not force the fact that you are right.

- Make it easy for the other person(s) to change their position without losing face (self-esteem).

- Express yourself in a serious, non-sarcastic manner.

- Offer multiple or alternative ideas or suggestions for developing a solution.

- If you are unable to stay calm and give rational feedback, postpone the discussion.

(SkillPath 1995)

Developing assertiveness

> *No one can make you feel inferior without your permission.*
> –Eleanor Roosevelt

One of the most important conflict-resolution skills is assertiveness. Do not confuse assertive behavior with aggressive behavior, which does not allow others to express themselves. Those who are assertive communicate in a direct and honest way and do not violate the other person's rights.

You will need to develop assertive communication skills so that when confronted by an "aggressor" you will be able to handle the situation as a professional. You know you are dealing with an aggressive personality when that person crosses the line and denies the rights of others.

 Tip: The key to being an assertive nurse is to be direct, clear, non-threatening, and non-attacking. Remember these tips when cultivating your own assertiveness skills:

1. You build confidence by believing in yourself. Think "I can handle anger," "I can deal with conflict," "I can deal with stress," and "I am confident." Repeat, rehearse, and visualize.

2. You must develop your communication skills through both verbal and nonverbal methods. Be mindful of your tone, volume, stance, etc.

3. You need to be prepared *mentally and factually* when dealing with others.

4. Saying "no" is a skill that you need to practice so that you do not cave in. It's okay to set limits and say no.

5. Handling disagreements involves allowing others to feel the way they do about an issue. Try using the "let's agree to disagree" approach. Everyone is entitled to his/her own opinion and it's okay if both of you do not reach an agreement. As long as you are both showing respect, your opinions do not need to match.

How to start a difficult discussion

You are having difficulty with a coworker and need to discuss it with her. You want to communicate effectively, but are unsure about how to approach the conversation.

So as to not trigger defensiveness in the other nurse, start the conversation off along these lines:

"I'm concerned about how we've been working together lately. I wanted to get your thoughts on this."

Then, continue the conversation using the "When you, I feel, I want" dialogue:

1. "When you . . . (address the behavior you want to discuss)"
2. "I feel . . . (identify your feelings)"
3. "Because . . . (list the effects of the behavior on you)"
4. "I'd like . . . (voice your desired solution/outcome)"

Practice this dialogue so that it comes naturally the next time you find your-self involved in a conflict.

Handling anger in others

When under attack by an angry person, there are several things you can do:

- Reflect on the message and acknowledge the person's issue. When dealing with an angry patient, for example, you can say, "I can see that you are upset that the test is overdue—let's talk about it."

- Take the conversation to a private place. Tell the person that "I do want to talk with you about this, but it needs to be in a private place."

- Repeat what the person has said. In this way, you can ensure that you are identifying their line of reasoning.

- Actively listen without interruption. The person may calm down once he/she knows that you are open to their needs.

- Respond with acceptance, such as, "I can see you are really upset about this."

- Offer to discuss a solution later and arrange a specific time to discuss it.

(SkillPath 1995)

Finally, remember that you are only responsible for your own behavior and emotions. If you feel that a situation is getting out of hand, don't be afraid to call in a third party, such as your manager. It is his/her job to assist and resolve problems on the unit.

Helpful Web sites

- *www.flylady.net*—Cleaning tips

- *www.webshots.com*—Photo organizing

- *www.stress.org*—American Institute of Stress

- *www.drweil.com*—Andrew Weil, MD's Web site on integrative medicine and self-healthcare.

- *www.mypryamid.gov*—Free nutrition counseling

- *www.self-esteem-nase.org*—National Association for Self-Esteem

- *www.sleepfoundation.org*—National Sleep Foundation

- *www.seedsofsimplicity.org*—Organization focused on simple living

- *www.mentalhealth.about.com/health/mentalhealth/cs/stressmanagement*—Stress-management resources

References

Adamson, Eve. 2002. *The Everything Stress Management Book: Practical ways to relax, be healthy, and maintain your sanity*. Avon, MA: Adams Media.

Aiken, L., et al. 2002. Hospital Nurse Staffing and Patient Mortality, Nurse Burnout, and Job Dissatisfaction. *Journal of the American Medical Association* 228: 1987–1993.

American Institute of Stress. 2006. What is Stress? *www.stress.org*.

Cherry, B., and S. Jacob. 2005. *Contemporary Nursing Issues, Trends, and Management*. St. Louis, MO: Elsevier Mosby.

Gill, J. 2003. *Stress Survival Guide*. NY: HarperTorch.

Marquis, B., and C. Huston. 2003. *Leadership Roles and Management Functions in Nursing: Theory and Application.* Philadelphia, PA: Lippincott, Williams and Wilkins.

Oregon Mediation Center, Inc. 2006. Effective mediation resources: Training Manual. *www.internetmediator.com/medres/.*

SkillPath Seminars. 1995. *Conflict Resolution and Confrontation Management.* Mission, KS.

Zerwekh, J., and J. Claborn. 2006. *Nursing Today: Transition and Trends.* St. Louis, MO: Saunders Elsevier.

Chapter 9

Legal pitfalls in nursing

The healthcare industry is constantly changing to meet fiscal and consumer demands. The work environment is changing, the patient population is changing, and the level of accountability expected by the public has heightened. These factors, among others, have led more and more nurses to be named as defendants in malpractice lawsuits. Nurses can be charged with negligence when a nurse fails to act in the best interest of the patient and violates a standard of nursing practice (Croke 2003).

In addition to the factors listed above, malpractice cases against nurses have increased due to

- the delegation to Unlicensed Assistive Personnel (UAP)

- early discharges of patients from hospitals

- the nursing shortage and increased hospital workload

- advances in technology

- increased autonomy and accountability of nurses

- informed consumers

- expanded legal definitions of liability (Croke 2003)

In her analysis of 350 case summaries, Eileen M. Croke, EdD, ANP, LNC-C, identified the six major categories that lead to malpractice lawsuits:

1. Not following standards of care
2. Failure to use equipment properly
3. Miscommunication or failure to communicate effectively
4. Documentation issues
5. Lack of assessment and monitoring
6. Failure to act as an advocate for the best interest of the patient

Ask: To avoid becoming one of the many nurses involved in legal turmoil, you need to understand the judicial system and how you can manage and reduce your risk of liability. And as a new graduate, now is the best time for you to learn about the legal pitfalls in nursing—as it's always better to be proactive than to be named in a legal suit.

Understanding law: The essentials

Legal definitions

Fact: In order to understand the legal system, there are several terms you first need to understand.

Tort law: A tort is a civil wrong for which the law allows the injured party to seek damages, or a remedy. It is a violation of some duty clearly set by the law and not by a specific agreement between two parties. It includes negligence and professional negligence.

Negligence: Conduct that falls below the standard established by law for the protection of others against unreasonable risk of harm. This includes the concept of "foreseeability" (i.e., that the harm that occurred could be anticipated). In nursing, negligence is measured by "the ordinary, reasonable, and prudent nurse" standard. JCAHO defines negligence as the "failure to use such care as a reasonably prudent and careful person would under similar circumstances."

Negligence by commission: When an individual does something that an ordinary, reasonable, and prudent person (i.e., another nurse), would not do.

Negligence by omission: When one fails to do something that is considered a "duty."

Professional negligence/malpractice: An action committed by a professional that falls below the professional standard of care. The JCAHO defines this as the "improper or unethical conduct or unreasonable lack of skill by a holder of a professional or official position."

Liability: Responsibility for an actual loss, evil, or burden, for which justice requires the individual to compensate the victim (Brent 2001).

What is needed to bring a case to trial?

There are four essential elements that must be proven for a patient to successfully bring a tort against a nurse to court:

1. **Duty:** the patient must show that the nurse had a duty to the patient.

2. **Breach of duty:** the patient must define what the appropriate standard of care was and show how the nurse violated that standard.

3. **Causation:** the patient must prove that this breach of duty caused the patient's injury.

4. **Damages or injuries:** the patient must prove that damages resulted because of the breach.

If those elements are satisfied, the case will likely head to trial. But before it does, the defendant will meet with an attorney who represents hospital employees. The attorney will prepare the defendant for a deposition, which is a way of getting testimony prior to court proceedings. If the defendant is a nurse, some of the following questions may be asked during the deposition:

- Did you successfully complete an orientation program before being assigned to provide care?

- Was a preceptor used for the orientation?

- Did you follow the patient-care policies and procedures?

- What does the most recent performance appraisal say about you? If there were areas needing improvement, did you follow through with the recommendations?

- When was the last nursing seminar or inservice program you attended?

Managing your risk

The legal risks for nurses are high. You are the front-line provider; in court, you will be held accountable under the state Nurse Practice Acts, national standards of nursing practice, and the care that you provided to your patient. You will have to demonstrate adequate competence and compliance with established organization policies. The care you provided will be evaluated by professional and state standards and a nurse expert.

Tip: No one ever wants to be placed in a situation of potential liability. To prevent a claim of professional negligence, you must

- follow established standards of care, facility policies, and procedures

- document all assessments and outcomes in a complete and timely manner

- identify any high-risk areas (i.e., areas where errors are commonly committed, such as failure to follow protocol, physician orders, or family complaints that have merit) and be vigilant about avoiding errors

- continually review nursing journals and nursing research to stay current with any changes in patient care

- keep up to date with any changes in unit or organization policies

- be aware of current nursing statutes and standards and comply with them

It's also important that you keep up with any expected competency and skills training needed for your job. Likewise, if there is any new equipment added on your unit, be sure to attend the inservice offered. If you are ever involved in a legal proceeding, your personnel file will be reviewed and you want to be sure your job orientation was completed and your annual competency and education requirements were maintained.

Caution: YOU are responsible for the care you delegate

Registered nurses are not only responsible for all of the care they provide, but also for the care they delegate. When you countersign patient-care flow sheets without truly assessing the situation for yourself, you leave yourself open to liability. A signed patient-care flow sheet indicates that the care was given within the standards and protocols for the organization. Unfortunately, however, nurses do not always understand the implications of their signature when working with licensed practical nurses and unlicensed assistive personnel.

Case study: Countersignature liability

A 90-year-old patient sustained a fall with fracture during an inpatient hospital stay. Based on the definition for a reportable event in that state, the director of quality assurance submitted a report. During the investigation, it was noted that the bed exit system did not alarm. In fact, it had been turned off. The patient had ambulated without assistance and thus had fallen, sustaining a fracture.

Subsequent to submitting the report to Department of Public Health (DPH), the director of quality assurance received a telephone call from DPH regarding the reportable event. In addition to inquiring whether additional remedies had been put in place as a result of the incident, the DPH surveyor asked the following questions:

- Why was the bed alarm off?

- Who was the last one to check the alarm?

- Who is responsible for ensuring the bed exit system is on for the patient's safety?

- What actions were taken to prevent this from happening to other patients?

These questions were all answered after a discussion with the nursing supervisor. However, in reviewing the patient flow sheet, the area for "bed alarm check" was checked off for every two hours—even though the unlicensed assistive person had not checked the bed alarm in the hour before the fall. The RN had countersigned the flow sheet, indicating that the task had been done, but in fact, it had not. Both the RN and unlicensed assistive person were counseled. The RN was reminded of the legal aspects of the clinical record and possible ramifications of the countersignature.

Moral of the story: **To minimize your risk, make sure you review those tasks you've delegated and ensure your documentation is accurate!** Remember, the best defense is always prevention.

Your documentation: Truth or consequences

Years ago, there was a game show called "Truth or Consequences." The clinical record can be very much like that game show. Either you have truth—i.e., everything you need to know about the clinical care of the patient in the medical record—or you face consequences—i.e., an accusation of substandard or poor-quality patient care.

The truth about truth

Let's start with the truth aspect of the clinical record. The clinical record needs to reflect an accurate and complete account of the care rendered. Like a book, the medical record should tell the story of the patient's care. It should have a beginning, middle, and end. Any reviewer who reads the medical record should get a good clinical picture of the events, care, and patient outcome. There should be no incomplete flow sheets and/or graphic sheets, or lapses in progress notes. It should include the right date, time, and clinical status, as well as the clinical care provided.

 Watch out: Many times in reviewing a clinical record, these simple items (e.g., date and time of assessment) are missing. Although it may seem inconsequential to the nurse, this missing piece may become critical in the court of law. Questions will undoubtedly be raised against the nurse, including:

- How can you prove that your documentation entry was timely?

- How do you prove that your assessment and intervention were based on the patient's condition at that time?

- What if those preceding you also did not document the date and time?

- Does this show a pattern of documentation that is unsafe?

- Does this demonstrate clinical documentation is not valued?

The medical record doesn't just convey the truth about the patient's care—it also illustrates the level of competence of the healthcare provider (you) and the truth about your commitment to safe, quality care. A complete medical record will

- tell the story of the patient's care

- reflect the documentation of high-quality, non-negligent, competent care

- serve as the best defense against allegations of negligence and fraud

Although nurses often view documentation as a dreaded task, healthcare professionals have a *legal duty* to maintain an accurate and complete medical record in sufficient detail.

Tips for documenting care

In an article in *The Journal of Perinatal and Neonatal Nursing,* authors Greenwald and Mondor offer several strategies for properly documenting care:

- Document all care given. This will be measured by the state Nurse Practice Act and standards of professional nursing practice. It is also proof that care was, in fact, given.

- Document any conversations with providers. Include highlights of the conversation, when the provider was notified, the response, instructions, and orders.

- Document any nursing interventions that occurred before and after notifying the provider.

- Never use the medical record as a battleground. Keep derogatory comments out of the medical record. Never blame another individual or department in the clinical record.

- If the chain of command was used, document the names of those contacted; the manner of communication; the time; the message communicated, and the response; any new orders given; and the patient's response to the newly ordered care.

- Always complete all forms/documentation tools.

- Document all sponge counts (OR, Labor and Delivery).

- Document patient instructions given, conversations held with the patient/family, and their level of understanding.

- Use only the accepted methods for correcting charting errors in the medical record. Check with your organization's policy.

- Do not document opinions. Stick to the facts (Greenwald and Mondor 2003).

In addition to the above tips, here are some bonus guidelines:

- Sign your name and credentials for every entry, even if it is just one line.

- Do not leave any blank spaces on your signature line. Draw a line through any remaining space to prevent forgery.

- Use black, permanent ink for entries. Do not use colored or felt tip pens, or pencils, as these do not copy well and may be easily altered.

- Never document a procedure or medication before it is administered.

- Use only abbreviations approved by the organization.

- Ensure the patient's correct name and identifiers appear on every medical record page.

- Do not countersign any order, narcotics count, narrative entry or other documentation unless you can attest to the accuracy of the information.

- Make an entry in the medical record whenever the patient leaves your care (e.g., for diagnostic testing work). Include the time and the condition of the patient upon leaving.

- Include the following information in the medical record when a patient is transferred: date and time of the transfer, patient condition at the time of transfer, who provided the transfer, where and to whom the patient was transferred, and the manner of the transfer.

- Document consent for or refusal of treatment in the record.

- Always use correct spelling, punctuation, and grammar.

- Never document for another person.

Facing the consequences

The consequences of an incomplete and inaccurate medical record leave the nurse and the organization vulnerable. Because various members of the healthcare team review the clinical record to ascertain the status and subsequent interventions needed for a patient, missing information may influence the practice of other professionals and consequently lead to multiple cases of professional liability.

Eight common charting errors

Accurate and complete nursing documentation is essential for demonstrating compliance with standards, delivering state-of-the-art nursing care, and communicating effectively with everyone involved in your patient's care. To avoid making errors in your own documentation, make yourself aware of these common charting errors and how to steer clear of committing them:

1. **Failure to document pertinent health or drug information.** To avoid this kind of mistake, you need to know how to take a thorough history. Be especially careful with patients who cannot communicate effectively (e.g., a poor historian, or dementia). It is important that conversations with family members, the transferring agency, or any other source of information be used. Also consider using bright labels and other accepted means to communicate the information.

2. **Failure to record nursing actions.** Here is where the rubber meets the road. To avoid leaving out essential actions, chart as close to the time as possible, even if it is only a one- or two-line entry. Also, reduce redundancy and chart facts once. You do not need to repeat the same information in more than one place. Just be sure it can be found in the clinical record.

3. **Failure to record medications given.** This may seem obvious, but how many times have you reviewed a Medication Administration Record (MAR) and found the previous shift's nurse said in his or her report that the patient had been medicated, but you could not find it documented in the medical record? Avoid nursing negligence by recording all medications given and the rationale for those not given, even if you may perceive them as insignificant. Always investigate when you suspect that a medication may have been administered but not recorded.

4. **Recording on the wrong chart.** Sometimes a simple mistake of misfiling can lead a nurse to chart on the wrong patient. Staff members are especially vulnerable to this error when patients with similar names are on the same unit, so you need a system of identification that is clear and as foolproof as possible. Always strive to ensure compliance with JCAHO's National Patient Safety Goal that refers to proper patient identification prior to procedures and medication administration.

Eight common charting errors (cont.)

5. **Failure to document a discontinued medication.** When a medication has been ordered to be discontinued, the change must be appropriately noted according to policy and communicated to the next shift's nurse. Nurses must comply with the organization's policies concerning "cross-checking" the physician orders with the MAR. Doing so can prevent serious complications.

6. **Failure to document drug reactions/changes in patient's condition.** The literature on "failure to rescue" points to this potential error. Nurses are responsible for the assessment of the patient's reaction to medication, or the identification of any change in the patient's condition. You must have the skill and knowledge to anticipate the clinical needs of the patient. You must also possess critical thinking skills to intervene appropriately in any adverse reaction or worsening of the patient's condition. But performing this assessment, identification, and intervention is not enough. You must also document that you have done so.

7. **Improper transcription of orders or transcription of improper orders.** The RN can be held liable for transcribing improper doses that led to a patient's injury. You can also be held liable if you transcribe and carry out an order that you know to be inaccurate or suspect as incorrect. If you discuss both the order and your concerns with physicians, document these conversations. In addition, if you maintain that administration of the medication or proceeding with a procedure is not in the best interest of the patient, activate the chain of command and document that as well.

8. **Illegible handwriting or incomplete records.** Illegible handwriting is no longer being tolerated by regulatory and accreditation surveyors. All providers who document in the clinical arena must ensure that what they have written is readable.

Handling documentation errors

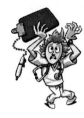

Don't panic: What happens if you make a documentation error? Do you know what the correct and accepted method of correction is? First, check with any existing policies or procedures regarding charting errors. If you cannot find anything in writing, call your risk manager. There should be established guidelines for you and your staff to follow.

In the past, we corrected any charting errors by writing the word "error" near the mistake. The standard today is to write "mistaken entry" above the line drawn through the words that need to be deleted. The author's date, time, and initials go above "mistaken entry."

Helpful hints for correcting errors

- **Keep the original entry intact.** Never scratch out or attempt to obliterate the previous entry. It gives the perception of trying to "cover up" and could cast doubt as to the integrity of the writer and the medical record. Just put a single line through the entry that needs to be changed with the time, date, and writer's name. In this way, the original entry can be read. Sometimes it is of benefit to write the reason for the correction such as "Mistaken entry, wrong medication name written."

- **Indicate late entries.** If a late entry is necessary, the writer should indicate such. For example: "8/24/06 2:30 p.m. Late entry for 8/24/06 10:00 a.m." The writer should then continue with the documentation that was intended for the earlier time.

- **Avoid altering numbers/words.** Never try to change a word or number into the correct one you intended. Handwriting experts may be asked to testify that the word/number was changed. This can give a false impression of fraud. It is best to just write "mistaken entry" and the reason, if there is room.

- **Make corrections promptly.** For example:

    ~~1/24/04 1320 Ambulated with assistance to BR. First void post delivery, clear yellow urine, no pain with voiding.~~
    ———————————————————————————————— P. Jones, RN ———

    1/24/04 1325 Mistaken entry above, charted on wrong patient.
    ——————————————————————————————— P. Jones, RN

Adverse events: When a bad thing happens

According to the Institute of Medicine's November 1999 report "To Err is Human: Building a Safer Health System," between 44,000 and 98,000 people die in hospitals each year due to preventable medical errors. Medical errors are defined as the "failure of a planned action to be completed as intended, or the use of a wrong plan to achieve an aim" (IOM 1999). Not only do such errors create public distrust, but they also cost healthcare facilities millions of dollars each year in litigation costs. The most common errors occur during the course of providing patient care. Examples include adverse drug events, improper transfusions, surgical injuries, wrong-site surgery, suicide, restraint-related death, falls, burns, pressure ulcers, and mistaken patient identity.

When an adverse event occurs, it is important to follow the organization's policy regarding responding, reporting, and recording. The policies of the organization will be reviewed by the Department of Public Health, the board of nurse examiners, and attorneys (if the case raises evidence of negligence). Your participation in ensuring accurate documentation in the medical record, accurate incident reporting, compliance with established policies, and assistance with the follow-up investigation is vital, especially in protecting you against culpability.

Ask: If an adverse event does occur, evaluate your risk by asking:

- Did I follow organization policies, procedures, and practices in this event?

- Did I check my nursing documentation for accuracy and completeness?

- Did I notify the necessary persons (e.g., the nurse manager or shift supervisor)?

Figure 9.1: "Do I need to report this?" quiz

Read each scenario. Circle "Y" if you believe the event needs to be reported and "N" if you do not.

1. During ambulation of a patient the patient hits the bedside table with his arm.   Y   N

2. Your PCA reports that a patient was found on the floor   Y   N

3. Shortly after administering a medication to your patient, you noted a mild reaction of a rash, itching, and skin warm to the touch.   Y   N

4. During a procedure, the equipment involved did not function properly   Y   N

5. Postpartum neurogenic bladder unresolved at discharge.   Y   N

[Answer key: All answers are yes.]

Defensive documentation: Where, what, when, and why

When an adverse event occurs, emotions are high and critical thinking may be clouded. Stay focused by thinking in terms of where, what, when, and why.

Where to document

Document your assessments, observations, interventions, and outcomes in the clinical record. An incident/occurrence report will also have to be completed. Do not refer to the incident report in your nursing progress notes.

What to document

Keep in mind that immediately following an adverse event, documentation may be reviewed by the quality and risk-management departments, the physician, the patient/family, and others. Also remember that what is written at the time of the event will have to stand on its own merit for five years. It may take that long for it to go through the legal process.

Ask: Read your documentation after it is written and ask yourself these questions:

- Is my documentation factual, objective, complete and as accurate (FOCA) as possible?

- Will it make sense to any reader?

- Do I have the accurate date, time, and sequence of events?

- Will I remember the intent of my documentation if called into question?

When to document

Don't forget: Did you document as closely as possible to the actual events as they occurred? Though you may be tired and stressed by the events that have occurred, the timing of your documentation is critical. You need to document the event and the required documentation elements as close to the time of the event as possible. Although late entries are an acceptable form of documentation, they may raise questions in the case of an adverse event.

Why to document

> *The palest ink is better than the strongest memory.*
> –Chinese proverb

Documentation needs to be *part* of patient care, not apart from it. The reason for your documentation is clear: our memory often fails us when put to the test in a malpractice case. In the case of an adverse event, the "why" to document is simple: **If it was documented, then it was done.**

Documenting the incident in the medical record

In many states, the incident report can be reviewed by the plaintiff's attorney, so methodical documentation here is also crucial. When documenting an incident, it should be a factual account of the incident, including treatment, the patient's response to the care, and any follow-up care that was provided. Also, if the patient or family stated something about their role in the incident, be sure to include it in both the incident report and the progress note. For example, if the patient stated, "I know you told me to ring the bell, but I thought I could do it alone," this may help the defense attorney prove that that patient contributed to the negligence. It would be said that the patient was guilty of contributory negligence (i.e., conduct that contributed to the patient's injuries) or comparative negligence (i.e., conduct that involves determining the percentage of each party's fault) (Weinstock et al. 1999).

Final thoughts

It's well known that nurses do not like to document—whether it's in paper or computer format—but proper documentation is the key to keeping yourself free and clear of legal repercussions.

 Click: The Nursing Services Organization has a great Web site you can check out to review legal cases that involved nurses. It will give you an idea of how skipping a simple nursing action could lead to legal nightmares. Check out their monthly-posted cases at *www.nso.com/case/cases.*

References

Brent, N. 2001. *Nurses and the Law.* Philadelphia, PA: WB Saunders Company.

Cahill, J. et al. 1992. *Nurse's Handbook of Law and Ethics.* Springhouse, PA: Springhouse Corporation.

Greenwald, L., and M. Mondor. 2003. Malpractice and the perinatal nurse. *Journal of Perinatal & Neonatal Nursing* 17(2): 101–110.

Institute of Medicine. 1999. To Err is Human: Building a Safer Health System. *www.iom.edu.*

Ladebauche, P. 2001. Lessons in liability for pediatric nurses. *Pediatric Nursing* 27(6): 581–588.

Joint Commission on the Accreditation of Healthcare Organizations. Glossary of terms. *www.jointcommission.org/sentinelevent/se_glossary.htm.*

Weinstock, D. et al. 1999. *Mastering Documentation.* Springhouse, PA: Springhouse Corp.

Chapter 10

Looking to the future

You made it

Your first year is over and you made it! You cannot put a price tag on the experiences you have had. If you look at what you have learned, it is incredible—you were able to pull your theoretical knowledge together with your experiential knowledge, you survived orientation, you figured out how to get along with your coworkers, and you learned how to manage your workload, among hundreds of other things. Yes, there were bumps in the road, as well as steep inclines, but you persevered and can now look back and triumphantly shout, "I made it!"

You have grown professionally and are beginning to move toward becoming a "proficient" nurse. You are only one year older, but you are so much wiser. The new graduate nurses will be looking to you for guidance and support. Do not let them down! Remember, we all started at the beginning and it is our responsibility to change the unhealthy patterns of behavior to positive ones.

What's next?

As you settle into the advanced-beginner stage of nursing, you can now concentrate on managing your professional and personal goals, and planning your financial future.

Professional goals may include advancing your education by completing your baccalaureate degree or starting your graduate work, getting your specialty certification, applying for a clinical nurse leader position on your unit, or moving from your current unit to a specialty unit, such as the trauma or intensive care unit.

Personal goals may include taking care of your own health or wellbeing, spending more time with old and new friends, and or moving to a new place. Whatever objectives you have identified for yourself, plan them well and stick to the plan. Nursing is an arduous but rewarding profession and taking care of professional and personal goals will be your lifeline.

Now is also the perfect time for you to start planning your financial future. Getting your finances in order as soon as possible will surely benefit you in the long run. And don't worry, once you understand the basics, you'll be well on your way to savings.

Professional development

Tip: Once you have settled into managing your job and yourself, you need to consider joining a professional organization. Aside from being recognized as someone committed to the profession, there are many perks to joining a professional organization:

- Networking opportunities (which help you when looking for other positions)

- Collegial support, especially during tough times

- The opportunity to learn about other facilities

- Access to news regarding current trends in nursing, as well as any political changes that may impact nursing practice state- or nation-wide

- Continuing education opportunities (often at a discounted rate)

- Invitations to national or state conventions

All of these opportunities will reenergize you and keep your passion for nursing alive. When you join a professional organization, you see the power of the collective voice. United, nurses have more knowledge, resources, and strength than any individual nurse could ever have. Think about staffing patterns, nursing practice standards, violence in the workplace, and workplace safety practices—who do you think monitors these issues? Professional organizations, of course.

The American Nurses Association (ANA) is the recognized professional organization in Washington, DC. They guard our scope of practice, look at how to improve our work environments, and protect the public by holding nursing to professional standards.

Aside from the ANA, there are a multitude of nursing organizations and associations you may want to consider joining. The following list comes from the National Institute of Nursing Research.

Nursing organizations
American Academy of Nursing
American Association of Colleges of Nursing
American Nurses Association
State Nurse Associations and Constituent Member Associations
International Council of Nurses Research Network
National League for Nursing
Sigma Theta Tau International, Inc.

Minority/ethnic nurses associations
Asian American/Pacific Islander Nurses Association, Inc.
National Alaska Native/American Indian Nurses Association, Inc.
National Association of Hispanic Nurses, Inc.
National Black Nurses Association, Inc.
National Coalition of Ethnic Minority Nurse Associations
Philippine Nurses Association of America, Inc.

Professional nursing and practice organizations
Academic Center for Evidence-Based Nursing
Academy of Medical Surgical Nurses
American Academy of Nurse Practitioners
American Assisted Living Nurses Association
American Association for the History of Nursing
American Association of Critical-Care Nurses

American Association of Diabetes Educators
American Association of Neuroscience Nurses
American College of Cardiovascular Nursing
American College of Nurse-Midwives
American College of Nurse Practitioners
American Nursing Informatics Association
American Organization of Nurse Executives
American Psychiatric Nurses Association
American Radiological Nurses Organization
American Society of Law, Medicine, and Ethics
American Society for Pain Management Nursing
American Society of Perianesthesia Nurses
Association of Child Neurology Nurses
Association of Rehabilitation Nurses
Association of Women's Health, Obstetric, & Neonatal Nurses
Emergency Nurses Association
Grounded Theory Institute
Hospice Patients Alliance: Consumer Advocates
International Society of Nurses in Genetics
International Society of Psychiatric–Mental Health Nurses
National Association of Bariatric Nurses
National Association of Clinical Nurse Specialists
National Association of Neonatal Nurses
National Council of State Boards of Nursing
National Gerontological Nursing Association
National Nursing Staff Development Organization
National Organization for Associate Degree Nursing
National Organization of Nurse Practitioner Faculties
Oncology Nursing Society
Society of Pediatric Nurses
Society for Vascular Nursing
Wound, Ostomy and Continence Nursing Society

Professional certification

In another year or so, you may think about pursuing professional specialty certification, which is granted by nursing organizations to those nurses who demonstrate an advanced level of competence. To earn your certification, you must complete a set number of clinical practice hours and pass a certification exam. When you become certified, you will add "RN, C" after your signature (in some hospitals, they allow the certification initials on your name badge).

The largest and most-well-known nursing credentialing program is the American Nurses Credentialing Center (ANCC), which is part of the American Nurses Association. The ANCC offers six specialty certification programs to all nurses with an associate's degree or higher: cardiac/vascular, gerontology, medical-surgical, pediatric, perinatal, and psychiatric and mental health. If you are interested in pursuing certification in another area, such as critical care, diabetes, gastroenterology, or wound/ostomy and continence care, check with the ANCC or that specialty's respective organization. These certifications often require a higher level of education or advanced degree.

Planning your financial future

Good money management is about adopting a healthy attitude toward money.
– Rebecca Knight

So you are finally making your own money, but are on the brink of drowning in student-loan and credit-card debt. What happened to the idea of earning money and spending it on fun things? Well, that idea is not completely out of reach—it just requires some planning.

Living beyond your means will lead you down the wrong path and to bad consequences. You need to get your money in order as soon as possible. Do not procrastinate and put it off until next year. That will only waste time and put you further in debt.

Get organized: Your life in a file folder

We have talked about staying organized in your work and home life. Now you will need to get organized in your financial life. Go out and buy an accordion-type file folder—one that is big enough to hold one year of expenses. Pick out a brightly colored one with tabs that you can mark as follows:

- Auto

- Credit cards

- Contributions

- Education

- Income

- Insurance

- Medical

- Mortgage/rent

- Taxes

- Utilities

- Miscellaneous

This is now your file for everything you will need for tax day. Put your paid bills and receipts in their respective slots. This file folder will also help you when planning your budget, as the things that you have paid for will be at your fingertips.

The National Endowment for Financial Education's "10 basic steps to getting smart about money"

1. Get organized.
2. Know where your money goes.
3. Shop smarter.
4. Look at your debt.
5. Reduce your debt.
6. Build a strong credit report.
7. Save for your future.
8. Set financial goals.
9. Create a spending plan.
10. Invest money to reach your goals.

The 3 Bs of finance: Budget, bank, and bargains

Budget

Most people hate the word "budget" just as much as the word "diet." But if you think of these terms in a positive light, they are both healthy living styles. Budgeting does not mean eliminating fun and the little extras in your life—it simply means planning them into your expenses.

Start out by tallying all of your expenses (see Figure 10.1). Be honest and account for *all* of your spending in the past month—that includes your daily coffee, take-out meals, and snack machine purchases. Look at your expenses in comparison to your income. Are your spending habits exceeding your monthly income? Don't stop this exercise now; you are just beginning to put yourself on the right track. You need to build yourself a realistic budget that will help you stay on track toward a strong financial future.

Figure 10.1: Personal financial plan

Personal financial plan
Year: _____

Net income.. $_____

Monthly expenses:
Savings (Pay yourself first)..................................$_____
Rent/mortgage...$_____
Property taxes..$_____
Heat...$_____
Electricity..$_____
Rent/mortgage insurance...................................$_____
Food...$_____
Car payment..$_____
Car insurance..$_____
Car repair/maintenance.....................................$_____
Gasoline..$_____
Phone/Internet/cable service...........................$_____
Cell phone..$_____
Life insurance..$_____

Other expenses:

_____ ....$_____

_____ ....$_____

Net income - monthly expenses =
Expendable income... $_____

Begin by looking at your priority spending, or those things that must be paid, like student loans, rent, utility bills, and food. Then look at your not-so-necessary expenses, like daily coffee or lunch expenses, and try opting for cheaper alternatives, like making your own coffee or bringing your lunch to work.

You will also need to look realistically at your recreational and clothing expenses. Your budget must account for all of these expenses, including your golfing fees and splurges at the mall. If you can help it, avoid using your credit card for these purchases—if you don't have your own money to cover the cost, do you really need to buy it? Remember you are looking at surviving your first years out of college. You must prioritize the "need-to-have" with the "nice-to-have" expenses.

There must also be a spot in your budget for savings. A lot of financial advice books recommend "paying yourself first." This is the secret to getting what you want and learning how to become a disciplined saver. Try your best to put some money, even if it is only a small amount, into a "rainy-day fund," otherwise known as a savings account. Life can take unexpected turns, and you need to be prepared.

Bank

Banks are vying for your business. Be sure to choose a bank with no fees attached to checking, savings, ATM, or online banking—those little fees add up!

Tip: The most efficient use of your time and the best way to stay ahead is to pay your bills online. Most service providers also allow you the option of electronic bill payment, a service which automatically deducts the bill amount from your bank account each pay period. This is especially helpful in managing your student loans, credit cards, and utility bills. If you use this service to pay off loans, however, try to set up the payment to deduct more than just the minimum amount due—that way, you'll pay off your debts quicker.

Why wait in line or worry about getting to the bank before it closes? Instead, have your paycheck automatically deposited into your account. If possible, set this up so that the majority of your paycheck goes into your checking account and the rest goes into your savings account. This is a painless way to start saving for your rainy-day fund.

Bargains

This is the word that my children always make fun of me for. I live by the motto "never pay full price for anything"—and that includes everything you know could be on sale at some point (grocery items, shoes, clothing, cars, etc). There is such a markup on all of those items. Why pay full price for clothing, for example, when you know that by mid-season it will be marked down and the store will also have a coupon for 15% off?

Tip: When shopping for groceries, look through your Sunday circulars and write out a list of what you need. Now find the store that has the best price for milk, juice, meat, etc. for that week. There will be a better price on each of those items each week, but you have to be willing to change name brands. Do not be embarrassed about clipping coupons or hunting for deals! Would you throw away five to 10 dollars in the garbage each week? Probably not, so why throw away coupon ads? Use that extra 10 dollars you saved for incidentals, or put it away for your next vacation's fun money.

Don't forget: The not-so-obvious bargains are those offered by your employer. If your organization offers flexible spending and/or retirement plans such as a 401(k) or 403(b), take advantage of these plans. They will not only save you money, but *make* you money as well.

Flex spending, as it's called, deducts money from your pre-tax dollars (i.e., your gross income) and puts that money into an account that you can draw from when you incur healthcare and/or childcare expenses. You save by not paying taxes on these expenses; so, for example, the next time you buy those new eyeglasses or need to fill a prescription, you won't have to worry about paying any tax.

Retirement plans are another great way to get started on the path to financial security. Under a 401(k) plan, you invest a certain amount of your income into your retirement account and your employer then contributes a certain percentage of money to your account as well. If you can afford to, put the maximum amount your employer will allow each month. If that's not possible, just put in whatever you can afford—in fact, why not try investing that money you saved from making your own coffee and brown-bagging your lunch?

Investment basics: The advantage of starting early

Here is a quick lesson in compound interest:

Let's say at 22 years of age you decide to put $2000/year (that's only $167/month, or $42/week, or $6/day) into a retirement/mutual fund that earns 9% interest. You stop making annual contributions to this fund when you are 30 years of age, when you have made an investment of $18,000. You do not contribute anything else. If you do not withdraw any money from this account, by the time you are 65 years of age you will have accumulated $579,471!

If you wait until you are 31 years of age and make annual contributions of $2,000 until you are 65, your total investment would be $70,000 but you would only have accumulated $470,249. When you look at the numbers, you start to understand the advantages of starting to save and invest early (National Endowment for Financial Education).

Long-term planning

If you are carrying credit-card debt, you need a long-term strategy to pay this off. Start by looking at your monthly credit-card interest rates and make sure that you are paying off as much as you can on the card that carries the highest interest rate. Always try to pay more than the minimum/expected amount.

Don't forget: If you are sinking in credit-card debt, call your credit-card companies and see if you can negotiate a lower monthly payment plan or lower interest rate. Remember, credit-card companies want your business, so they are often willing to negotiate with you.

Good debt versus bad debt

First, let's define good debt and bad debt. Put simply, good debt is the kind of debt where, over time, you get something back for all the money you spent and sacrifices you made. Buying a home and paying a mortgage is an example of good debt. As you know, houses appreciate in value over time and are considered a good investment.

Watch out: Bad debt, on the other hand, is the kind of debt where, after your money is spent, you have nothing left to show for it. Buying a car or carrying balances on your credit cards are examples of bad debt. Of course, you need a car for transportation, but after the car is paid off, it's quite likely that, sooner or later, you'll need another one. Remember, cars do not become more valuable over time but rather lose their value.

Consider Don and Lisa, a young couple in their mid-20s. They both wanted to buy a house but didn't think that they could afford this big step. They spoke with a realtor regarding what it would cost to buy a small, starter home and found that they would not be able to afford the monthly payments. Don and Lisa continued to grow frustrated about renting, knowing that this would not provide them with any equity or increase their wealth.

One day at a family gathering Don was sharing his frustration with his relatives. His aunt noticed that both he and Lisa owned new vehicles. So she asked, "What do you both pay each month for those cars?" Their monthly payments were $1,500.

The answer was obvious now: sell the new, expensive cars, buy used cars, and start using the extra cash as a down payment for a house. Lesson learned: Don and Lisa could increase their personal wealth by buying a home and building equity (good debt) **only if** they were willing to forego driving new, very expensive vehicles that over time would become less valuable (bad debt).

The 3 Rs of money: Reality, responsibility, and restraint

Reality: Recognize that unless you strike it rich, which is highly unlikely, you will have limited amounts of time and money to use.

Responsibility: If you handle your money wisely, you can do a lot of good for yourself and others. But, it's your own fault if you blow your money.

Restraint: Learn delayed gratification. Have the self-control to save your money for a future goal instead of spending it now (National Endowment for Financial Education).

Don't forget: Having the life you dream about does not just happen by accident. It requires planning. You have reached your goal of becoming a nurse by following a strict academic plan and sticking with it—secure your financial future by doing the same!

Helpful Web sites

- *www.cccsintl.org*—Consumer Counseling Service (provides budget counseling, educational programs, and debt-management assistance)

- *www.grocerygame.com*—Printable grocery coupons

- *www.IHatefinancialplanning.com*

- *www.moneymanagement.org*—Financial guidance, free credit counseling, and debt-management assistance

- *www.myvesta.org*—Credit and financial assistance

- *www.nefe.org*—National Endowment for Financial Education (provides budget counseling, educational materials, and debt-management assistance)

Final words of wisdom

- You can't (and shouldn't) know everything. Ask questions.

- Remember the business aspect of healthcare. Ask yourself: Is this clinical decision a good business decision?

- Your mentors will change as you grow.

- Have two hobbies that you love—one that is physical (and keeps you fit) and one that is not (something you can do even as you age).

- Critical thinking is a necessity for survival in healthcare. It will increase with age and experience.

- One of the best aspects of the nursing profession is all the opportunities it offers. Take full advantage of them.

- Patients will leave their mark in your heart; some will even help you to balance your life.

- You will touch another human's life in a way that no one outside of the profession will understand.

- Hearing the words "thank you" from a patient will make it all worthwhile, even on your worst day.

- You will learn something new every day; treasure it.

- Join your state nursing association, and be an active participant.

- You are a teacher of health—educate!

- Do not judge your patients; advocate for them.

- Stop to visit or say goodbye to your patients at the end of your day. You will put a smile on their face and give them confidence in the care they receive.

- It's normal to cry.

- Don't become the victim of physician abuse.

- Join a committee to improve patient outcomes.

- Remember, the nurse is the patient's last defense against poor-quality care.

- Recognize when you are in a toxic environment and escape.

- Accept constructive criticism as part of the growing process.

- Take responsibility.

- Use humor to get through the tough times.

- Keep smiling; it takes less effort than frowning.

- Realize how fortunate you are to be the one giving care instead of receiving it.

- Be a lifelong learner (McNamara 1999).

References

Knight, R. 2003. *A Car, Some Cash, and a Place to Crash: The Only Post-College Survival Guide You'll Ever Need.* Emmaus, PA: Rodale.

McNamara, R. 1999. *Welcome to the World of Everyday Heroes: Tips for Thriving in Your First Years of Nursing Practice.* Wolcott, CT: Kelsco Press.

National Endowment for Financial Education. 2006. 3 R's of Money: Reality, Responsibility and Restraint. *www.nefe.org/hsfppportal/files/11240_Step%20Four.pdf.*

National Endowment for Financial Education. 2006. 10 Basic Steps to Getting Smart About Money. *www.smartaboutmoney.org/nefe/pages/content.asp?page=1300.*